# TAOIST YOGA

An ancient system of energy utilization for improving mental
and physical vigour and combating stress.

*By the same author*
THE TAO OF LONG LIFE

# TAOIST YOGA
## The Chinese Art of K'ai Men

*by*

CHEE SOO

THE AQUARIAN PRESS
Wellingborough, Northamptonshire

First published 1977
First Trade Paperback Edition (revised) 1983

British Library Cataloguing in Publication Data

Soo, Chee
    Taoist yoga: the Chinese art of K'ai men.
    1. K'ai men
    I. Title
    613.7      RA781.7

    ISBN 0-85030-323-0

The Aquarian Press is part of the
Thorsons Publishing Group

Printed and bound in Great Britain

# Contents

|  | | Page |
|---|---|---|
| 1. | Introduction | 9 |
| 2. | The Path of K'ai Men | 13 |
| 3. | The Sections of K'ai Men | 21 |
| 4. | The Importance of Good Health | 36 |
| 5. | Breath is Life | 42 |
| 6. | Hints for Good Practice | 53 |
| 7. | Postures | 60 |
| 8. | Movement with Stillness | 69 |
| 9. | Meditation | 150 |
| 10. | Healing | 155 |
|  | *The Chinese Cultural Arts Association* | 158 |
|  | *Index* | 159 |

# Acknowledgements

I would like to express my gratitude to Chris Wuesthoff, John Solagabade, Diane Wright and Dorothy Hargrave for the time and help they gave in the preparation of this book.

Chee Soo

## Chapter 1

# Introduction

Many Westerners are under the impression that the Chinese do things back to front or the wrong way round. Agreed, the front of a Chinese book, for instance, is what in the West would be the back, and the Chinese read from top to bottom instead of from left to right. This, however, has to do with the type of script being used. Neither the Chinese nor the Western method is any "better", or more logical, than the other.

In other fields too, though, the Chinese have always maintained what may seem to Westerners to be a back-to-front approach. If spots suddenly appear on his skin, a Chinese does not rub ointment onto them to make them disappear, and then watch them come back another day. He does not take a pill to ease a migraine attack one day, only to have to go through the same routine again the week after. Instead, he goes to the cause and root of the trouble, tackles it, and so seeks to put paid to it for good. The Chinese have followed this principle throughout their very long history.

In the period 10,000-3,000 BC, which is generally known as the Primitive Period (Yuan Shi She Hui), the Chinese were very, very superstitious, and this led them to explore the depths of the supernatural, spiritualism, physical and spiritual alchemy, psychic forces, the spheres of the occult, the many directions and channels of the mind, the different pathways in meditation, and the vast and different energies and vitalities that exist within ourselves and within all phenomena in the universe. This vastly increased their understanding of these things, into which they delved far more deeply than any Westerners have ever done.

Every aspect of psychic research was minutely studied and scrutinized, in every conceivable way, so that the human body became an "open door". To begin with; the universe seemed, to the Chinese, like a baby that they tried to bring to maturity through understanding themselves. But, in understanding themselves even more, they realized that they were the babies and that the universe was their mother.

In addition, the enormous energies and vitalities of all things within the universe were given minute and painstaking research. The existence and properties of macro-cosmic and micro-cosmic energies were explored, and it was realized that these vitalities abound in the human body, as well as in everything else. It was this that eventually led the Chinese to formulate the concept of the Yin and Yang and of Dual Monism.

The basic ideas of the "lines of meridian", which are extensively used in acupuncture, meridian healing, spot pressing, vibration healing, Li healing, Ch'i healing and Chinese massage, were formulated during this period. Originally they were used to open up the psychic and energy centres of the human body, and even to this day they are still used in this way. However, greater emphasis is now placed on their uses in healing.

Meditation, with all its various outlets and channels, was thoroughly explored, and principles and rituals were laid down so that all could follow the pathways without losing their way. Healing by meditation was also discovered, and enormous advances were made in the understanding of herbs and herbal therapy. Ancient Chinese records contain details of over 30,000 different herbs.

The so-called "Primitive Period" was thus a dynamic and progressive era in every field, but mainly in the understanding of spiritual matters. Divination, spiritualism, superstitions, the exploration of the supernatural, utilization of colours, numerology, the study of natural forces and so on were studied to such a degree that no avenue was left unexplored and no stone left unturned in the endeavour to understand the principles on which the universe operates and what it is that makes each person tick.

In the period from about 3,000 BC to about the time when Jesus Christ was born, the principal Chinese moral, religious and philosophical systems were laid down. This was the time of the great Chinese thinkers and saw the formation of numerous religious groups, many of which survived for only a comparatively short while. Others, however, such as Taoism and Ch'an Buddhism, went from strength to strength and still flourish today.

There are many Westerners who believe that Taoism is just an old, and now outdated, religion. Such people, who, like as not, are so earthbound that they can see no further than the car parked outside their house, or the clothes they wear, or the mortgage they have wrapped around their lives for years to come, or the ill health they suffer, day in and day out, are to be pitied, for the truth is that Taoism is as alive today as it was thousands of years ago. This is thanks to the teachers who have perpetuated it in their own lives and through communicating their experience, insight, and understanding of the Tao to others.

Many of the sages of the period 3,000 BC to 1 BC wrote down their thoughts, beliefs and admonitions, but time, wars and so on have caused many writings to be lost or burnt. However, China is fortunate in that a goodly number of the writings of Lao Tzu, Chuang Tzu and Confucius are still available, even though they are not always translated according to the true Chinese trend of thought. There are many Western authors who, not being Taoists, have tried to create an impression of mystery about the Tao, and to make it sound weird and out of this world. At the root of Taoism, however, lies a very simple belief in the balance of the opposing, but complementary, forces of Yin and Yang, and the harmony of Dual Monism, so that, whilst being separate, everything is one within the universe, and all are one with the Supreme Spirit of God, if you want to give it a name.

From about 1,000 BC, the Chinese began to pay greater attention to the physical and cultural sides of their lives, and to explore in great depth physical alchemy. At about the time that Bodhidharma went to the Shaolin Temple — about 200 BC — the martial arts began to be developed. To begin with, they were very, very hard and vicious, using sheer brute force and muscular strength, but, as the practitioners of these arts became

aware of how to control and use their internal energy (Neichung
Ch'i), so they learned how to take direct blows by fist or
weapons without feeling the slightest pain and without being
marked at all at the point of impact. The monks who trained at
the Shaolin Temple in those days became very well known for
the very hard physical training that they had to endure daily.
They also became renowned for their prowess at boxing.

Back in the Primitive Period, eight basic physical exercises —
most of them exercises from a sitting or squatting position —
had been devised and developed to help open the channels of the
body and the mind to spiritual awareness. Bodhidharma
increased the number of basic stances to eighteen, most of the
new ones being exercises from a standing position.

At about the time when Christ was born, the emphasis moved
from the "exterior", or "external", arts, based on hard physical
prowess, to the softer, "internal" arts. Great emphasis was
placed on using the internal energy as an outward force, beyond
the sphere of the body, and physical pliability, flexibility and
softness of mind and body became the key to exploration of the
self. It was during this period in Chinese history that the art of
T'ai Chi Ch'uan, with thirteen basic stances, was first
introduced, and that K'ai Men, Taoist yoga, developed, and
became part of the Chinese way of life. Initially it used the eight
basic stances mentioned earlier.

Thus, in developing their understanding of the universe and
themselves, the Chinese began at the true beginning, by
exploring the spiritual world; then, turning to themselves, they
concentrated their endeavours on the code of ethics and their
morality, and from there went on to develop their religious
beliefs and philosophical outlook; and, finally, they completed
the circle by looking closely at the body, its health, the energies
and vitalities that exist within it, and the way in which these can
be cultivated, harnessed, controlled, and utilized to benefit
others. Westerners may seek to use physical exercise as a way of
opening up the way to the mind and the spirit, but, as K'ai Men
and all other parts of Taoism emphasize, the true beginning is
with the spirit itself. Only by beginning in this way can one
expect to reach a real understanding of the forces in the universe
and in the self, and to see things as they really are.

## Chapter 2

# The Path of K'ai Men

Taoist yoga has long been known as the "Open Door" (K'ai Men), although at various times in its long history it has also been referred to as Ho Ping ("Unity") and Ho Hsieh ("Harmony"). K'ai Men is the most appropriate name, however, as it expresses the idea that Taoist yoga is the doorway to all the channels of the mind, the spirit and the body. All these, while retaining their separate identity, are as one, so reflecting the balance of Yin and Yang and the Dual Monism of all in the universe.

As outlined in the previous chapter, the foundations of Taoism, and, thus, of K'ai Men itself, were laid down in the Primitive Period of Chinese history. During that period, the first golden rules for all Taoists to follow were laid down, and one of the most fundamental of these was *"Never harass, never hinder, never harm and never hurt anyone, either by thought or by deed."* Living and thinking this is hard, but the good sense and morality of it are undeniable.

Do fish in the water complain that it is cold or dirty? Of course not. Do they complain because the sea becomes rough, or envy or try to exploit each other? No. They live in harmony constantly, never envying or hating anything. Life for them is simply living. There are no comparisons in nature, and even love is meaningless outside the world of mankind.

It is living now that matters. The way to the spirit is through constant good thoughts and good deeds, *now and every minute of each day*, and through this way of life everything becomes an "open door" and the Tao becomes apparent to you in everything you do, and in every thought that passes through your head.

As the very first step towards attaining full control of yourself and deepening your consciousness and awareness, your must purify the internal and physical side of your life by sensible eating and drinking habits. Eating the Ch'ang Ming way (see Chapter 4) will purify your internal organs, bring you good health, and so make you feel fitter and more relaxed than you have ever been before. In following this course, it matters not what your religion might be, for Taoism is not a religion — not even a belief or a trend of thought — for it is the pathway, the road, the track, of your own way of life, which was laid down for you long before you were ever born. Have the good sense to follow it, have the initiative to learn, have the understanding to exercise control, and be aware not only of what is going on around you, but also, and most important, of what is going on inside yourself.

Having got on to the path of sensible eating and drinking, so learning to behave as a part of nature and become closer to it, the next step for you to take is to aid the energies of your own body to realize their true potential. These energies fall into four very simple categories.

## 1. Physical Energy
The physical energy of your body is utilized through the muscles and tissues of your anatomy, so that, when, for instance, you lift something, these automatically come into effect. In K'ai Men we call these "muscle changes" and it is through muscle changes within the body that the exercises of K'ai Men are most effective. Through the muscles of the body we begin to open up the channels that are necessary steps towards opening every door within us. Good eating and drinking habits help towards this by making the tissue of the body more flexible, and, whilst you slowly grow older in years, they still remain young in their texture. Revitalizing the body comes not only through our daily eating habits but also by specialized and constant deep breathing exercises, which not only help the normal channels to attain added vigour, but also assist the psychic channels of the body to be opened and strengthened.

In addition to the muscular system, we also have within us an intricate system of blood vessels, which takes the goodness to every part of the body. It is aided by a complex nervous system. Whilst being separate in their specialized fields they all operate as one within the human frame. In addition to sensible eating and drinking habits, to make the body even healthier, to gain vitality, and to assist in the cleansing of the whole system, it is essential to have an adequate supply of oxygen. So deep breathing constantly is also a must for the purification and energizing of the body.

## 2. Mental Energy

To enable the mind to be the constant link with the spirit, passing messages back and forwards, to have it in constant control of every thought, every emotion, every sense, and every action of the body and limbs, no matter how minute that movement might be, you will readily understand that it requires enormous energy. It is when the mind becomes depleted of vitality and energy that you begin to feel listless and tired. Concentration itself burns up terrific amounts of energy, so, if you seriously want to meditate, ensure that your body has the energy and vitalities within it to be able to feed the mind in accordance with all its needs and requirements. Good and proper eating and drinking habits, coupled with constant and regular deep breathing every minute of your life, are therefore a *must*.

## 3. Internal Energy

Apart from the physical and mental energies of the body, we have what is commonly known as "internal energy" (Neichung Ch'i) or, more technically, as "intrinsic energy" (T'ien Jan Neng Li), but most people who practise the Chinese arts call it the "vitality power" (Sheng Ch'i). One of the objectives of all those who practice the Chinese arts is to arouse, cultivate, develop and control its dynamic force. There is nothing mysterious about it, for it is the natural energy of the body, and everyone is born with it. You see this power come into action when, for instance, a little baby grips your finger. It has not had time to develop any muscles, yet it will grip your finger so tightly that you may wonder how it could do so. Unfortunately, when you reach five or six years of age you begin using your physical strength so much that your internal energy or vitality power becomes almost dormant, and you use very little of it as you grow older.

This natural power of your body enables you to do your everyday work without the use of physical strength, and without running yourself down and becoming tired and listless. Have you noticed how weary and run down you seem to get round about October and November of each year? This is because you have just entered a Yin period of the year, which always affects the muscles, tissues and bones of the body. If you rely too much on the physical side of your body to do your daily work, you will certainly feel the strain.

Internal energy helps to revitalize the various functional, control and psychic centres within the body so that they not only become more supple and flexible, but also become more receptive. In addition to this, it enables you to meditate much more strongly, because the mind has an unlimited source of energy that it can call upon at any time, whenever it requires it. This energy is built up through many various breathing exercises. All of these have specific jobs to do, but their main task is to heat up the Lower Stove or Cauldron (Hsia Lu) or Golden Stove (Chin Lu), as it is referred to in Taoism, which lies in a position about thirty-four millimetres below the navel. The heat so generated creates and activates the vitality force.

The benefit that the body derives from this power is beyond normal appreciation and comprehension, but in its own way it fights bacteria within the body and your body health improves enormously, so that colds and influenza, along with other complaints, become things of the past. Most Westerners, however, if confronted by a demonstration of the dynamic power of internal energy, would rather explain it away as hypnotism, or whatever, than believe the evidence of their eyes.

This vitality power is so powerful that with the use of it almost everything is possible: a woman might withstand forty or fifty men pushing against one of her hands. Besides improving the health of the human body, and one's physical powers, this vitality power helps the lift-off of your spirit when you die, and, if you desire to meditate whether internally (mentally) or externally (spiritually), this internal power will enable you to transmit or transport to the furthermost paths of the spiritual world. Without this energy, meditation will be a failure. Many people have travelled the whole world trying to seriously meditate, yet so many come back to the point from where they started disillusioned and disappointed — only to find that what they were looking for was within themselves all the time, and that they need not have taken a single step outside their door to find it.

## 4. Macro-cosmic Energy

The other source of energy that is vital to our own personal lives is "macro-cosmic energy" (Ching Sheng Li), which was a part of your life before you left your mother's womb. This energy comes down from the heavens, passes through all Yang things, with a centripetal circular motion, and enters the earth, where it gathers further vitality. It then returns to heaven, passing through all Yin things, with a centrifugal circular action. The general movement of the energy is thus as follows:

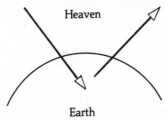

In passing through Yang things on its way to earth, it passes through man — down his spine and out from his abdomen. Conversely, in passing through Yin things on its way back to heaven, it passes through woman — up her spine, round the head and out through the mouth. The two directions may be represented as follows:

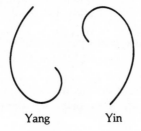

If you put the two together, the result is the famous Yin and Yang symbol of China, representing the unity and duality, the Dual Monism, of all things.

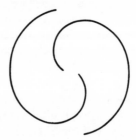

Our bodies, the persons that we are, the food that we eat, the water that we drink, and even the illnesses that we suffer all depend on the balance or unbalance of Yin and Yang. Mentally, physically and spiritually everything is governed by these two simple elements, and nothing is totally one or the other, though some things are predominately Ying or Yang.

Macro-cosmic energy is everywhere, and it passes through you constantly. If you learn to store it, harness it, control it and learn to mix it with your vitality power you can reach the realms of immortality. This source of energy enabled many of the sages and philosophers of ancient China to live to 150 to 200 years of age, and Lao Tzu is said by some to have lived for over 300 years here on earth. But you too can join us in the knowledge that age is only the number of earth years, and at sixty you can still have the skin, the mind and the energy and vitality that you had when you were twenty. Time is nothing; it is how you use it, live it and utilize it that really matters, and your present life and your spiritual growth depend on it. Don't let precious days slip by wasted; learn to live properly, and attain some physical, mental and spiritual satisfaction in your life, and seriously take up the study of K'ai Men, so as to learn what makes you tick, and how all the energies of the body can be utilized and strengthened. There is an open door, just walk in, and start learning a little bit more about yourself.

When you have built up the internal and external energies of your body, you can then begin to develop your spiritual control, consciousness and understanding. To have this control of oneself, you must start with your way of living, always thinking good, doing good, and never harassing, hindering, harming or hurting anyone, by word, by thought or by deed, and learning to serve others here on earth, and the Supreme Spirit (God).

First of all try and understand yourself every minute of every day, and try not to make any comparisons at any time. Remember that there is nothing good, and nothing bad, for it is only humans who always try and set standards by making one thing a bit better than another, or make it worse by comparing it with something else. There are no comparisons in nature. All things are equal, and we are all exactly the same, and no one or no thing is any better or worse than something else, no matter how or what or why we live from day to day.

The material things of life, the Rolls Royces, the big diamonds, the beautiful clothes, are nothing, but nothing will stop you buying them if your concern is to show others how well of you are, or that you are better than they. But remember seriously that you were born with nothing and will die with nothing, and so learn to live with nothing. In so doing you will find that all things will be found for you, and you will never have to make a decision; never have to worry about this or that; and never even give a second thought to how you are going to survive. This is the Tao, a way of life that, once you have learned to accept it, will show you how wonderful life is and how beautiful is nature, of which we all are an integral part. So try to understand the Tao, try to be a part of it constantly, and in so doing try very hard to understand and appreciate all of it within yourself.

If you scratch your hand, or stub your toe, or if you drop something, then immediately stop to think back within the last thirty seconds or one minute, and try and collect your thoughts and remember if you had a bad thought during this time, because this could possibly be what we know in Taoism as the Law of Repercussion (Yin K'uo). If you do something more serious — that is, harass or harm somebody — then you can guarantee that someone will be doing the same to you, if not quite in the same way, within a very short space of time. So learn to try and understand it, endeavour to see it and in so doing learn to appreciate it. Then your eyes will be opened and you will begin to see the Tao. This understanding takes time, but, if you get into the habit of turning your thoughts inwards, you will start to understand the outward sphere of things that happen in your life every day.

The violence in this world is only what we make it ourselves; these are the repercussions of our own deeds. There is no danger for those who truly live the way of the Tao, because if you think no evil, and do no evil, then evil will not exist.

When we no longer think of good deeds and good thoughts, then even goodness disappears. When we no longer see bad thoughts and bad deeds, then badness itself will disappear. When we no longer compare one with another then all disappear, and we understand the Tao.

Say your prayers regularly, whatever your religion; say them morning, noon and night. You are a part of the spiritual world, it is a part of you, we are *one* and, although we seem separate in our physical, earthly bodies, this is nonetheless true. To realize this and think along these lines is the beginning of spiritual growth, spiritual maturity, spiritual advancement within yourself, and this is the true understanding of the spiritual world, of which we are an integral part.

This is the object of the "Open Door" (K'ai Men) through the physical exercises, which will enable the whole of the body to be opened and therefore become more receptive; through the specialized breathing exercises, which will help to strengthen and revitalize the various channels and centres within our human body, which will establish the links with the mind; and through our thoughts and our deeds, which will open the way to our spiritual growth, our advancement, and our spiritual maturity. This is the true path of the Open Door, which never closes, yet many never try to open it at all.

When you have done all these things and lived the way of the Tao and have tried to understand it, become conscious of it, aware of it to the point of becoming enlightened, then, having made this circuit, you will come back to the beginning. You will have made the complete circle of the Yin and Yang of the physical, the mental and the spiritual, and will come back to the very commencement of all things — namely, yourself.

## Chapter 3

# The Sections of K'ai Men

The Yang expansion of the spiritual, mental and physical in ancient China took place over about 10,000 years, up till the time of Christ. Over that period there was an enormous amount of exploration and experimentation, and as a result vast understanding was accrued. All the paths, channels and centres of the human body, the mind, the energies and the spirit became known, and this laid the early foundations of the Taoist belief and codes of living, showing how, by cultivating and activating all one's potentialities, one could eventually achieve the Supreme Ultimate, where one's personal spirit becomes united with the Supreme Spirit, or God.

To reach this ultimate goal takes many lifetimes, and during those lives we must have conquered ourselves in every way, to such a degree that we attain complete and utter unity within ourselves. When each individual section has reached such a degree of perfection that we have complete union and harmony within ourselves, then all can truly be combined to take the journey along the one road that leads to our heavenly home.

There are five "openings" (K'ou) or "doorways" (Men K'ou), which comprise the main sections of K'ai Men. These are (1) spirit, (2) mind, (3) body, (4) energies and (5) healing. Each of these sections has many subsections or "steps" (Pu), and every step that we take within a section will enable us to attain unity and harmony within it.

## Spirit

To be at one with your own spirit you must acquire a complete understanding of the universe, by appreciating and being conscious of the Tao and the path that you have been pre-destined to take in this life. Understanding this will give you a much clearer picture of your destiny on earth, and the way that you have to follow in your daily life. Being more conscious of the Tao will give you a deeper insight and concentration, not only concerning yourself, but also concerning other people. Through this consciousness you then become more and more aware of the Tao, and the work of the Supreme Spirit and see his work, and the results of his work, every day of your life.

You will also understand and appreciate that miracles happen every minute of every day, and that they are visible to anyone whose eyes are open to perceive them. Unfortunately, the average person in the street is so earthbound that he cannot see any further than the car he sits in, the glass he holds in his hand, or the mortgage on his house; and so his life is in continual conflict, because he is forever striving after money, and not after spiritual gain. If he but realized it, all things are found for those who live by the laws of the universe and the spirit, and as a result they need never worry about any of the mundane things of life. When you are close to your mother she will provide and protect you all the time, but when you are close to the Supreme Spirit you will be mothered as you have never known it before; all worries will disappear, stress become a forgotten word, accidents never happen; you will have well-nigh unbelievable good health, and life will be peaceful, tranquil and harmonious — like being in heaven, here on earth.

Changes are inevitable, because everything in the universe is on the move, and through constant movement changes, however slight, are continually taking place within and outside all phenomena. Therefore, by understanding the Yin and the Yang of the insubstantial as well as the substantial, you will be able to harmonize the spiritual side of your life with the actions of your body. When the physical side of your life is in close harmony with the spiritual side, you can then walk constantly with the Tao, and not only will your requirements be catered for, but all decisions will be made for you, and you will be protected night and day.

The Tao is the mother of all, and it is so very unfortunate that so many of her children here on earth are blind and deaf to so much, talk rubbish, curse and swear, and discuss only those earthly things they either love or hate, and have lost the taste of the true nectar of life. This misuse of the senses robs the body of a lot of vital energy, creates resistance to the wishes of the Tao, and retards the spiritual growth of the individual.

This spiritual growth is known as Taoist alchemy. Many Western authors have ridiculed the Taoists of ancient China and the thousands of years that they spent in their search for immortality — spiritual, mental and physical. Even now, writers are still talking of "Taoist mysteries" or the "mystic Taoists", and there is much debate about whether the great Taoist writers, notably Chuang Tzu and Lao Tzu, really existed, and, if so, when, where and for how long. Does it matter? Of course it doesn't, for the words that were written give such a deep understanding of the Taoist way of life that they will live on for all eternity. Such literature explains Taoism and all it stood for and continues to stand for. Even so, the true Taoist will find words quite inadequate, for nothing can replace actually living in accordance with the laws of the Supreme Spirit within the universe, and that is Taoism. It sounds simple and it is simple; it is only human beings who make things complicated.

Admittedly the Taoists went through many periods of vast experimentation and in almost every conceivable field. They explored every cranny in their search for something they knew existed, but, in those very early days, did not have the faintest idea how it could be obtained. So experiments continued over 10,000 years, until eventually the answer was found. When that happened it was realized that there was no question to answer, for the key to everything lies in one golden rule: *"Recognize the Tao and in so doing you will be able to live in accordance with the fundamental laws of the universe."* Through following this simple rule, everything is known, everything is understood, and therefore questions are unnecessary, and the whole of life here on earth and in the celestial sphere becomes an open book for all to see and to read.

This applies, too, to every phenomenon in the universe, for there are no secrets, no mysteries, and the reason why this is so is that everything created and controlled by the Tao is completely natural within itself and within its own sphere, for it abides by the basic foundations of the universal laws of its creator.

This same law applies to every human being, for we are also children of the universe, and, if we abide by the simple basic laws that have been laid down, our life is serene, uncomplicated, free from worry, hate, jealousy and lust, and we can travel on a sea of tranquillity every minute of every day. This is peace on earth. This is heaven on earth. This is the Tao. This is understanding.

So belief and understanding are the first two steps towards spiritual attainment and perpetual growth. Taoist alchemy also teaches the cultivation of macro-cosmic energy (see Chapter 2), which is the external energy of the body and the spiritual energy that comes down from heaven and enters all phenomena in the universe. It is the energy that enabled Jesus Christ to walk on the sea of Galilee and enabled him to rise from the dead, and it is the energy that enables your spirit to rise to heaven when your earthly body ceases to function. It is also the power that helps you to become reincarnated for your next life here on earth. So building up the receptivity of your body to this energy is absolutely essential, and this can be learned through Taoist alchemy. It teaches you how to harness, store, and utilize this energy, not only for everyday use, but also to build it up to such a dynamic force that it can be used for healing (for various energies can be used in many different ways) and will eventually ensure your passage to heaven.

## Mind

This section contains many subsections, each of which requires separate attention, so that it will aid and harmonize with the others, until eventually they all become one.

Physical purification is accomplished by eating the Ch'ang Ming way (see next chapter), for this certainly helps the circulation and tissues within the brain, and soothes and calms the nervous system so that there is more peace and tranquillity in the mind and the thoughts, leading to more positive thinking and better control. Changing your eating and drinking habits goes a long way towards giving you better and stronger control over your physical actions and more concentrated mental control; and through the change purification of the bloodstream takes place, which in turn cleanses the blood and tissues within the brain.

Mental purification is achieved by thinking good all the time, not letting in even one bad thought, no matter what is said or done against you, and no matter what you see. Accept everything that comes, remembering that it is not your place to judge; only the Supreme Spirit has the right, and, if he has arranged for such and such a thing to happen, so be it: it may be a just retribution. Never tell a lie, be open and frank all the time, for the truth is the Tao, and if you live by the laws of the universe it is absolutely unnecessary to try and hide something that has been so arranged on your behalf. Constant acceptance and truthfulness effect the purification of your deepest inner mind.

Acceptance includes acceptance of the laws of nature, so that the truth of everything may impress itself on the mind and you learn to accept graciously, without complaint or thoughts of changing it, everything that happens along the way without any thoughts pervading the brain on how you could alter it, or wishing that you could change it, or complaining that it is not acceptable. Accept the truth of life every minute of every day, whether it suits you or not, and no matter whom it involves. Learn to accept everything on its face value, even though it does not always seem to make sense to you at the time.

Good walks with the good, and it attracts goodness like a magnet, to the benefit of all concerned. If you think good and do good, at every opportunity, you will find that in the long run it will have the tendency to rub off, and others will feel your influence and eventually change within themselves, and in so doing they will become better people. When you set the example, then sooner or later others will automatically strive to follow.

Egoism should not be a part of your make-up. Be happy with what you have, even if it is a suit in tatters and a wooden box to sit on, for even that was given to you by the Tao, and remember you could have been in a worse state by having no suit and no box. Don't strive needlessly every day for something better; do your best at work or at home within your capabilities, and once the Tao sees that you are a dedicated person and have attained control over yourself and your mind, and that you have become a true child of the universe, then, and only then, will you see the benefits that the Tao can bring. If you already own a big house, and have money, use those goods to help in whatever way you can, for the Tao gave them to you in the first place. You can rest assured that what is given away is always replaced, unless it has been stolen or gained by fraud or violent means. Anything you have gained thus you may expect to lose, and, the greater the suffering and trouble you caused in gaining it, the greater will be your own misfortune in losing it. Remember that we are all spirits locked within a human body, and we are all a part of the Supreme Spirit, so indirectly we are all brothers and sisters. Therefore let us treat each other as members of a large and happy family. We are all spirits, all equal, and that should promote harmony amongst us all. If you are not happy with equality and wish for something better, you are living in a world of dreams and your ego is your boss; for, whatever you aspire to be, you cannot alter or change your spiritual sphere. Be happy with what you have, or the job that you do, and let the Tao do the rest of the planning for you.

Emotions are the outcome of stress in mind and in the body. When they oppose or react against each other, there is enormous stress, and emotions then come to the fore, and the safety valve of control loses its effectiveness and things start to happen. When the two harmonize or work together there is tranquillity and a unity of body and mind. With the mind constantly in control, there is no room for reactions, for the body is then kept properly in check.

Concentration is essential if you want to ensure that the mind is in constant control, and if you wish to meditate properly and sincerely then concentration is imperative. It is so easy to say you ought to do this or do that, but we all know how difficult it is when we are faced with the daily problems of living, earning a livelihood, and looking after a family. Concentrating in a quiet room on your own is certainly one way of improving control over the mind, but it is not the best answer to the problem, for in the time you do not spend thus you run the risk of undoing your progress. The best tip, and one that my own master gave me when I was still a teenager, was to learn to concentrate on each task in hand, no matter what it might be, giving it your wholehearted attention and allowing no other thoughts to enter your mind whilst you are occupied with the job you are doing.

This is the best way to concentrate, for it gets you into the habit of concentrating all of the time, not just for a few minutes each day. I took the tip that my master gave me and have found that it has really paid off, since I no longer have to think about self control.

Meditation is something that many would like to do, and many travel the world trying to find someone who can give them the key to the answer, so that they can transcend the everyday at any time they wish and reach a point of peace and tranquillity. If this is all that meditation means to you, then give up, for that is just egoism and it has no place in the spiritual world; or, if you are a sceptic about the next world and the part that our own spirit plays within the universe, then don't bother to try and meditate, for your mind and your spirit will not leave your earthbound body, and you will be just wasting your time, for you will drain what little energy you have in other directions, and will not have sufficient vitality to raise the mind beyond the level of your own skull. In any case, the gates of the celestial sphere will be opened only to those who sincerely believe, have managed to conquer their emotions and egoism, and are meditating for the right reasons. The portals of heaven are not open to every Tom, Dick or Harry who wishes to spy or look around for curiosity's sake. The reasons for meditating have got to be real and from the heart, and the person has to believe and acknowledge the Supreme Spirit, and have learnt to abide by the laws of the universe within himself.

Meditation is not just a matter of closing the eyes and then allowing the mind to wander off into space all on its own. You have to be in charge, for you are the driver and it is essential that you are in complete control at all times. In K'ai Men we learn how to drive properly, for we have over twenty ways of meditating, not only with the eyes closed, but also with them open. Complete control means constant concentration — you cannot afford to take your thoughts off the road for one second, or you will not succeed in meditating successfully. All this requires strong self-discipline of mind, body and spirit, and the build-up of the energies and vitalities of the body.

It is no good contemplating a very long journey without ensuring that you have sufficient fuel for the trip. With meditation this means enough for the initial take-off, which is the hardest part, and for the whole of the journey there and back as well. That is why it is a *must* to develop the vitalities of the body and mind, and it is one of the main reasons why Taoists pay particular attention to the cultivation, harnessing and control of such energies, which are so necessary to the human body in every way. The correct utilization of such energies, and the purpose for which they are used, are of primary importance too.

In addition to the energy centres within the head, there are also psychic centres, which are also developed to a very fine degree. These enable you to become hypersensitive and to feel vibrations and atmosphere more easily, acquiring a deeper insight not only into other people but also into the spiritual world. The senses become very acute and you become more and more aware of the development and growth of your internal true self, as opposed to your external self, which is purely an illusion consisting of pride, emotions, and vanity. The separation of one self from the other is the liberation of the individual, and the true Way becomes apparent, and awareness becomes reality, as the hurdles and barriers of the human self are cleared and swept away.

The first objective of meditating is to become a "no self", where self takes a back seat and illusions are erased from the mind, so that everything about the self becomes completely impersonal, and concentration and contemplation take over control. The mind has to be obedient if you are going to be successful in your meditation, and you have to control and train it and make it abide by the laws of nature, so that it will automatically activate and become steadily stronger as each day goes by. The process admittedly is slow, so regular and constant practice is necessary, to prevent emotional stresses, illusions and so on from permeating the inner mind. Whatever you do, try and take it nice and easy, don't let there be any strain or stress at any time, and don't push yourself in an endeavour to get quick results, for you can work only to the speed at which your mind can adapt. Your greatest enemy will be your own thoughts, for the disturbance that they cause can be most upsetting at times. Many pupils are discouraged by the difficulty they have in putting their mind in order, and therefore lose patience with themselves and give up, though very close to becoming positive in their concentration. A really good teacher is a great asset, for he can advise and help you in your persistent struggle for mastery over yourself, and can give you the guidelines that will enable you to avoid misdirecting your efforts. When you have succeeded in conquering the first stage, you will find that concentration will no longer be necessary, for obedience will be instantaneous, and you will pass through the thin dividing line between concentration and contemplation and find the door to meditation open in front of you.

Additional aids to the success of your meditation can be obtained through a more positive mind when practising the K'ai Men physical exercises, feeling the sensations that your body goes through, the muscle changes that take place, and the flow of your internal energy from one movement to another. These will help you to build up the control and concentration of your physical actions in conjunction with the mind, and will assist in your mental awareness as well.

K'ai Men will assist you to control your mind through thought, hearing, sight, smell and touch, all of which can be brought under strict supervision through constant practice. This will eventually make it possible for you to direct instantly the energies and vitalities of the body, open and close at will the numerous psychic centres, and utilize fully, for the benefit of all, the extensive healing powers of K'ai Men.

There are many ways of meditating in Taoism, and, whilst these can be listed as twenty basic paths, they are much subdivided, making the field of Taoist meditation very large indeed. Yet, because of the balance of Yin and Yang, it is highly contractile as well as enormously expansive, for it allows us both to explore deep within ourselves and others, and to travel from one end of the world to the other, and transcend the astral plane, the celestial sphere, and the heavenly orbit.

Even if you have reached the stage when you can fully meditate at any time that you wish, and in any field that you choose, you may progress yet further by exploring how to meditate with the eyes open. We call this "visual transportation" (Shih Li Yun Shu), in addition to which there is "spiritual transportation" (Ching Shen Yun Shu): both are very advanced stages of deep meditation, and thus very few have ever heard of them.

# Body

The human body is so intricate, and has so many channels and outlets, that it takes even a very dedicated person a long time to acquire complete control of it and internal harmony. Nevertheless, with a strong mind and deep concentration the Way will be found much easier.

The first stage is to purify the body, and this is done simply by accepting and abiding by the principles of Ch'ang Ming, the Taoist long-life therapy (see next chapter). Within approximately ten to fourteen days you will begin to feel the effect and benefits of the change, and at the end of a month to six weeks you will certainly see the difference as well. Thereafter any weaknesses that may previously have developed in the body will slowly be cured, and don't worry if you lose weight, for you will come down to your natural body weight. Those who are already slim or thin may not like the idea that they may lose some more weight, but don't worry, you will slowly regain internal health and strength and the weight your body settles at will be the right one for you.

The basic principles of Ch'ang Ming not only entail a complete internal purification, but also ensure constant good health thereafter, day in and day out, all the year round. Of course, like everything else that is really worthwhile, it will take some time to achieve fully, especially if initially these are weaknesses in the body structure or organs, so aim at about three years for a complete internal purification, especially if your eating and drinking habits have been typically Western. Certain adjustments will definitely have to be made in your private life — for instance, in the context of what your family eats.

External purification of the body is through the normal process of washing, showering and bathing, but be careful not to overdo the use of soap and bath salts, for too much use and they enter the pores of the skin and get into the bloodstream. If you have ever noticed that, if you happen to change the brand of soap you use, you break out in spots, you will realize the truth of this. The use of commercial Epsom salts in your bath water is one way of really purifying the external part of your body. It is sold by most chemists, and if you put two tumblerfuls in your bath (remembering not to use any soap or water-softener at all) you will not only cleanse your body thoroughly, but also feel extremely relaxed — so much so that it is wise to go straight to bed afterwards, for you will sleep like a log.

Through K'ai Men postures and exercises (see later chapters) you will attain physical suppleness and dexterity, and a state of physical fitness that will amaze you. The exercises can be practised at home as well as in the classroom, and can be accomplished by anyone, of any age, without stress or strain. They will help give you full control over your body.

## Energies

The normal man in the street does not realize how important energy and vitality are to the human body. It is only lack of energy in certain organs that causes illness and sickness, so, if your body is correctly energized throughout, and you constantly maintain the Yin and Yang balance, illness will be something that happens not to you, but to others, if they are ignorant of the workings of the human body.

Harmonizing all the energies within the body is something that K'ai Men will teach you to do. All phenomena in the universe consist of energy, and the vibrations they give off can be weak or strong, and either short or long. The energies of the body have to be built up so that they become stronger and stronger each day, and this can easily be accomplished by eating the correct food, executing the right breathing exercises, and seeing that you reach and maintain the correct physical balance.

The energy of the mind will be built up by the breathing exercises that you do, and the extra oxygen that these put into the bloodstream will enable the mind to do its work with greater zest and more dynamic concentration.

The various energies are described in Chapter 2.

## Healing

From time immemorial the Taoists have always been healers, endeavouring to harmonize the Yin and the Yang in every direction — spiritually, mentally, physically and through the energies and vitalities that influence our lives and everything within the universe. The continuous fluctuations and inter-actions of this negative-positive Dual Monism, as it is called, gave rise to the principles of the "five elements" (Wu Hsing), from which all actions, events and phenomena are derived.

The "five elements" are wood, fire, earth, metal and water, and the ancient Taoists plotted two diagrams showing the inter-relations of these elements: the Ho-T'u, showing the inter-connecting links in Yang sequence, which is the life growth of everything in nature; and the Lo-Shu, displaying these same elements in their Yin order, which is the destructive influence they have on each other when opposed. It is this understanding that enables all Taoists to appreciate every aspect of the human being — spiritual, mental and physical — and therefore to understand the various weaknesses that arise and how to cure them.

In the early spiritual era of China, Taoists learnt that prayer and incantations could cure, not only locally but also from afar, and through these incantations they learnt that vibrations could heal as well. By making use of the "lines of meridian" in the human body, both these methods were used successfully, and continue to be so used. Healing by meditation came into being during the same period.

Thousands of talismans were used by the early Taoists in their work, and many of them in that far distant era were able to project these emblems around themselves to heal and protect within the cosmic field in which they were working at the time. To the average Westerner it may seem that this was in some way occult, but there was nothing mystical or magical about it, certainly not as far as the Taoist is concerned. It also created harmony between phenomena through the field of inactivity, which in turn provided a very strong link between Taoist belief and Taoist philosophy. Today the Taoist wears only one emblem (which certainly will not be made of gold or gold-plated) and this is it:

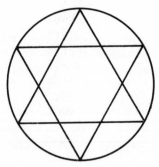

It is Dual Monism (the interlocking triangles), which represents the Yin and Yang of all phenomena in the universe (the circle). The six points symbolize the five elements and spiritual or macro-cosmic energy. It also shows the direction of flow of this energy from heaven and earth, and from earth back to heaven. The circle round the Dual Monism represents not only the universe, but also the void, which is the Tao. So the complete symbol stands for everything within and outside the cosmos — heaven and earth, the whole of nature and humanity, and all phenomena, known and unknown. All are one. Unfortunately, we know no Taoist who uses the art of the talisman today, and so possibly another ancient art of the Chinese has been lost in the annals of time.

Positive understanding of the Yin and Yang also gave the Taoists an insight into the vibrations and the strength of energy from various types of food, but it was only through thousands of years of experimentation that full knowledge was eventually gained. At one time they ate nothing but meat; at another only seafood; at another nothing but rice; then only grain foods; and so on and so forth. As a result of this fantastic dedication to experiment, it was found how to attain a perfect balance in one's eating habits, and as a result Ch'ang Ming (Taoist long-life therapy) came into being. It is still carried on today, thanks to the work of the Lee family over the last few thousand years, and particularly to Chan Lee, who showed how the therapy could be adapted to Western eating habits. As a result Ch'ang Ming is now available to all who want to obtain the correct balance of Yin and Yang in their own bodies and attain constant good health, so greatly increasing their chances of longevity. Living thus, their bodily energies will increase to such a degree that weariness and tiredness will no longer be a part of their lives, and they will find that there are not enough hours in the day to do everything they want to do, for they will have vitality to spare.

Herbalism is another field in which the Taoists excelled, and they explored this so extensively that they acquired knowledge of over 30,000 herbs. Herbalists abounded everywhere and would make up prescriptions on request, serving herb tea to waiting customers.

Even in modern China the ancient traditional remedies are widely used, alongside Western medicines, so today China is

getting the very best of both worlds. Many universities and
hospitals teach the old methods, and there are ten times more
doctors of traditional than of modern medicine in China.
Results show that this has not been to the detriment of the
nation's health.

Those taking up K'ai Men will learn many aspects of
herbalism, for, by balancing the Yin and Yang within the human
anatomy, herbs can bring about very quick recoveries from
illness. Centuries ago, Chinese herbs were carried along the Silk
Road, through India and Persia to Asia Minor and Egypt, and
ships constantly carried herbs from Peking, Hangchow, and
Macao across the Indian Ocean to ports on the Persian Gulf, so
great was the demand from the countries bordering the Mediter-
ranean. Even now, vast quantities of herbs are being trans-
ported all over the world, and one of the biggest sellers is
ginseng.

Ch'i and Li healing, which utilize the natural energy of the
body and the macro-cosmic energy of the universe, can be used
in healing and helping others, through the lines of meridian. The
principles are similar to those in acupuncture. The great
difference is that, whereas acupuncture uses various sizes and
lengths of needles, in Ch'i and Li healing the fingers and palms
are used to cause the lines of meridian to vibrate and thereby
transmit either Ch'i (internal) or Li (macro-cosmic) energy to the
points of weakness within the patient. Whilst this may sound
simple enough, it does require an ability to generate the various
energies as and when and to the degree needed; a knowledge of
how to read the pulse and of the principles of the Yin and Yang; a
full appreciation of the harmony and opposition of the five
elements; and an intimate knowledge of the lines of meridian as
laid down in the *Nei Ching* (the internal medicine canon; see
next chapter). To acquire the requisite ability and knowledge
requires serious, concentrated study, over a long period. It
requires too a first-class teacher (Chinese, ideally) to impart
these skills.

Now that the main sections of K'ai Men have been outlined, it
must again be emphasized that each has to be harmonized with
the others. In this way, you personally will be able to reach the
Supreme Ultimate, and you will be able to help, heal and serve

so many who are less fortunate than you. This is the Yin and Yang of your own personal life; this is the "open door" to the true concept of living; this is the understanding, the belief, and the philosophy of the Tao.

So the ultimate aim of all people who practise K'ai Men is to attain the supreme level of the physical, the mind, and the spirit, so that each can live as long as possible here on earth in this present life, to do good, think good, and help and assist other people on every possible occasion and thereby live in accordance with the divine laws of nature and the Supreme Spirit, hoping that others will follow that example and themselves follow the true path of their lives.

There are many rules of conduct as well as many rules of thought, but the following two Taoist guidelines should be remembered and observed at all times:

1. Think good, do good every minute of every day, and learn to help others as much as possible without thought of thanks or possible reward.
2. Never hinder, never harass, never harm and never hurt anyone, either by thought or by deed.

By abiding by these two rules of the Taoist, you will be assured that the Tao will be made known to you, and your eyes will eventually be opened, and then you will have the full understanding of the flow of nature and appreciate the work of the Supreme and Universal Spirit.

Abiding by these rules in your daily life, and through the regular practice of K'ai Men, you can energize and open every channel within the body, mind and spirit, so that you will not only feel the dynamic benefits yourself, but be able to help those with whom you come in contact.

All the doors to yourself are there already; all you have to do is learn to open them. Why not start *now*?

*Chapter 4*

# The Importance of Good Health

Why do we eat? Is it because we are hungry or like the flavour of certain things, or do we eat just for the sake of eating — clock-watching in other words? Lunch is at one, tea at five, dinner at eight, and it becomes a ritual, whether we need the food or not, and whether we are hungry or not. Because of this, few people realize the importance of eating and drinking correctly, and never fully appreciate that most illnesses are caused through bad and senseless eating and drinking habits.

Eating is essential to us, of course, and the pleasure of eating is important too, but we should all understand that the whole of our life revolves around our food intake and breathing, which matter to us not only physically but also mentally and spiritually. Through correct eating habits and learning to understand what is and what is not good for us, we can ensure that the body maintains constant good health, and that we grow older without looking old or feeling or being old within ourselves. Many sages of ancient China lived to be 130 to 200 years old, which in itself is a great encouragement to cultivate the correct eating habits.

Proper eating enables the bones, tissues and organs of the body to remain strong and healthy, and so ensures that the Yin and Yang are in balance within the body, and that ill health is foreign to it. For this to be the result, it is necessary to take into account not only the type of food eaten, but also when it is eaten and how it is chewed and digested.

17. Sea salt.
18. Seaweed and other sea vegetables.
19. Soya sauce.
20. Sesame salt.
21. Noodles.
22. Herbs.

*Processed foods.* Stay away from all foods that contain chemical additives (artificial colourings, flavourings, preservatives, and the like), none of which do the body any good. They tend, too, to make food too Yin or too Yang, which is to be avoided at all costs.

*Fruit.* Though apples are Yang, fruit comes within the general category of being Yin, and should therefore be eaten in very small quantities. Especially stay away from all tropical fruits, such as oranges, figs, pineapples, avocados, papayas, mangoes and bananas, for they are very Yin indeed. A woman who has been eating the Ch'ang Ming way for about three years, is pregnant, and at some time eats some tropical fruit and consumes two or three pints of liquid may suffer a miscarriage from no other cause than that. Anyone who happens to be ill should not eat fruit at all, and it is quite wrong to give fruit as a present to invalids.

*Vegetables.* Use only those that are locally grown and that happen to be in season at the time. If they are organically grown, then that is better still. Pulses, such as peas, beans and lentils, are especially good, since they are rich in protein, iron and many vitamins.

*Herbs.* Though herbs tend not to be used to the extent they once were, they are cheap and very useful. There are many, such as sage, thyme, parsley, mint, dandelion, burdock, basil, and bay leaf, that can be added to food and soups, and they all have excellent qualities. A number too, can be used to make drinks (for instance, mint tea, and dandelion tea and coffee).

*Rice.* White rice has been polished, and in some cases bleached, so it is much better to buy brown rice, which, though it takes a

little longer to cook, does retain its vitamins, which are
normally lost in processing. The short-grain variety is the best.

*Seaweed.* Seaweed is rich in minerals, proteins, vitamins and
enzymes. It can be eaten all the year round, and there is a wide
variety of different types available, many of them very
delicious.

*Grains.* Brown rice, barley, wheat, oats, millet, maize, rye and
other types of grain are valuable for producing energy and may
be consumed in a wide variety of ways: for example, as
breakfast cereal; in bread, cakes, biscuits, waffles, and so on;
and as the basis of various beverages. By browning grain in a
frying-pan, then adding water and boiling the mixture, a very
pleasant drink can be made (adding a little honey or soya sauce
to taste).

*Fish.* Once a week is more than often enough to eat fish, and this
applies to other seafood as well, such as shrimps, prawns,
oysters and crab. This is because these are all Yin foods.
Especially stay away from salmon, mackerel, swordfish and
shark (i.e. red and blue fish), which are extremely Yin.

*Meats.* Eat no red or blue meats (for instance, lamb, veal and
beef) and no pork, snails, rabbit or similar meats. Poultry and
game-birds may be eaten, but meat is by no means essential,
since all the nourishment the body needs may be obtained from
grain foods and vegetables.
     Most meat is, of course, full of chemicals from the foodstuffs
that the animals are given to eat, the fertilizers used on the land,
the antibiotics put into the animals by the vet, and the dyes,
colouring and preservatives added by man after the animal has
been slaughtered. In addition to all that, meat is very difficult for
the stomach to digest, since the fat and gristle content over-
works the digestive organs, and the toxins take a long time to get
out of the circulatory system, so putting a great strain upon it.

*Potatoes, tomatoes, aubergines.* These are distant cousins of the
deadly nightshade, share some of its properties, and so are best
left well alone.

*Salt.* Ordinary rock salt contains little or no goodness what-soever, but sea salt (which is much stronger tasting) contains various minerals and traces of iodine. Anyone fifty or more years old should consume less salt than a person of under fifty.

*Sesame salt.* This is normally referred to as sesame-seed salt and not only very tasty sprinkled over food, but also very nourishing. It is made up of one part salt to ten parts sesame seeds. First roast the salt; then roast the seeds until they begin to pop; and, finally, mix the two together and grind them (with a mallet and pestle or a pepper-mill) into powder.

*Coffee, chocolate, teas.* It is about time that people became more fully aware of the harmful effects of coffee and ordinary tea. They both contain caffeine, tannin and many other harmful ingredients, and because they also act as a stimulant they throw added strain upon the heart. Chocolate, on the other hand, is prolific in oxalic acid, which is a cause of acne in children and reduces the amount of calcium entering their bodies.

*Chewing.* To take some of the strain away from the digestive organs, chew your food really well — about fifty to a hundred times per mouthful. If you can make each mouthful turn into water before swallowing, this will benefit your health enormously.

*Chapter 5*

# Breath is Life

Breathing is accepted as the most natural thing in the world, but very few people really consider how important to the body correct breathing is. We can all go without food and water for many days, yet, if we stop breathing for even thirty seconds, we quickly realize that we cannot do without air for even a short while. Yes, we accept breathing without ever giving it a serious thought, unless we have the misfortune to suffer a complaint such as hay fever, asthma or emphysema, when breathing becomes really difficult.

Through bad habits or ignorance, the majority of people breathe very shallowly, using only about one-third of their lung capacity on each breath intake. Owing to this, their health is likely to deteriorate — fatigue, sluggishness, tiredness, headaches, bronchial complaints, wheeziness in the throat, and so on, becoming the order of each day for them. Lack of oxygen can throw an undue strain on the heart and create many circulation problems, which in turn will affect the tissues and bone structure, decrease sexuality, and affect the glands, the whole nervous system, and all internal organs.

Let us look at one or two of the complaints that people may suffer from mainly owing to poor or inadequate breathing.

Emphysema, a complaint that is now widespread, though virtually unknown before the turn of the century, has now increased, and every day sees an increase in the numbers that are suffering from this simple complaint. What happens is some of the tissues within the lungs dilate and become fused together, cutting down the surface area, and thereby causing the breathing to become more rapid. This throws an added burden on to the heart, which may fail if subjected to too great a strain.

Bronchitis, which is accompanied by a persistent bad cough, is generally the result of bad eating habits and too much fluid within the body. By correcting the diet and learning to breathe deeply and correctly, this simple Yin complaint can be eliminated.

Asthma can readily be recognized by the laboured breathing of the sufferer. It is caused by overworking of the kidneys and can be cured by breathing properly and limiting the fluid intake.

Many other illnesses too, including tuberculosis, pneumonia, hay fever, pleurisy and sinus trouble, are caused by bad eating habits and unsufficient oxygen in the bloodstream. When our lives depend so much on correct breathing, it is clearly imperative that we should learn to breathe properly, so that we are constantly in good physical condition and therefore in good health.

It is very important, at all times, to have sufficient fresh air entering the lungs, so that the impure blood in the body can be cleansed and purified through the action of the oxygen coming into contact with the blood within the lungs. If this purification does not take place, then waste products re-enter the bloodstream and the blood deteriorates, causing a general weakening of the body. Energies become depleted, making the body less resistant to illness and disease, and causing fatigue, which is the commonest cause of ill health. Learn, therefore, to breathe deeply every minute of the day, and eat and drink the Ch'ang Ming way, as described in the previous chapter. Correct and controlled breathing helps to open the channels to the psychic centres, revitalize and re-energize the body, and so open the way to the mind and spiritual development.

In the Chinese art of K'ai Men there are twenty basic specialized breathing exercises: eight Yin, eight Yang, and four a mixture of the two. Each of these has a specific job to do — some of them acting as a sedative, some as a tonic, and some assisting with the harnessing, activation and cultivation of the internal and macro-cosmic energies, and opening up the functional and control channels that feed and activate the energy and psychic centres within the anatomy.

There are two main ways of breathing, and these are each divided into two halves, each of which has three centres. The two main ways are Yin and Yang, but these each contain something relating to the other, as will be outlined below.

## Yin

Yin breathing is very shallow breathing indeed, and is the way that most people usually breathe. It is very unhealthy and is the cause of many chest, throat and head ailments. It raises the upper chest, shoulders and collarbone when an in-breath is taken, and is generally known as clavicular breathing. Because it causes pressure against the diaphragm, the lungs get very little air, and this means that the benefit to the blood and the body as a whole is very slight.

One of the variants of Yin breathing involves inhaling strongly and for longer than you exhale for, but be careful if you attempt this: it causes a very light sensation within the upper chest and head, and may make you feel a little dizzy. This is because Yin breathing stimulates the mid-brain, and increases the amount of energy attracted from the earth.

The Yin Micro-cosmic Orbit, or Inner Ch'i Circling, is another of the specialized Taoist techniques. By breathing deeply through the lower abdomen (Tan T'ien — the Lower Cauldron or Stove) — and using special arm movements in co-operation with a partner, the student can learn how to lock his internal energy or vitality power into the five positions indicated on Diagram 1.

The Yang Macro-cosmic Circle, Yin section, or Outer Ch'i Circle, is a dynamic breathing exercise that requires many years of practice at K'ai Men before it can even be attempted. This is because it demands a very strong Ch'i action, a dynamic depth of concentration within oneself, and positive mind control. The basic principle of the technique (see Diagram 2) is to breathe without taking an in- or out-breath (as usually understood), and it is accomplished through the soles of the feet, the middle of the spine and the top of the head. The internal energy is circled through these points and also out to the finger-tips. Only students who have spent many years practising all aspects of K'ai Men will fully appreciate what this means and how it is accomplished.

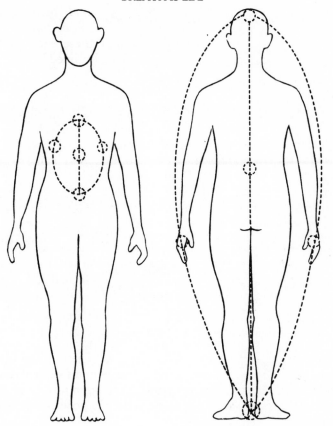

Diagram 1 Yin Micro-cosmic
Orbit, Yin section

Diagram 2 Yang Macro-cosmic
Circle, Yin section

## Yang

Yang breathing is very deep breathing because it concentrates
on the utilization of the diaphragm. In the West it is generally
known as diaphragmatic breathing. This way of breathing gives
greater freedom to the lungs and so their absorption becomes
more, but, because of the downward pressure on the abdominal
organs, which gives them an internal massage, the abdomen is
pushed outward. All this is stimulating to the lower abdomen
and increases the amount of energy attracted from heaven.

Another Yang way of breathing is to make your in-breath

short and sharp, but exhale strongly and for as long as you can. This method of breathing is the best for your health, for it helps to generate enormous energy, gives the blood all the oxygen that it needs, purifies the blood by the absorption of waste matter, and helps to strengthen the nervous system and give health to the rest of the anatomy.

The Yin Micro-cosmic Orbit, Yang section, combines the vitality power, or internal energy, with macro-cosmic energy. Through specialized breathing techniques these energies are raised as shown in Diagram 3: from point A up the spine to point E, at the top of the head. Both energies can be locked into the positions marked B, C, D, and E on the diagram, and these are known as the channels of control, which not only give positive and dynamic energy to the body and mind, but also vibrate the psychic centres and open up and strengthen the channel to the spirit.

The Yang Macro-cosmic Circle in the Yang section is the completion of the entire circle, from point E back to point A, through F, G, and H, and after completion of the full circle the energies are controlled back to the lower abdomen or lower cauldron, where they are harnessed and revitalized. The openings from point E down the front of the body to point A are known as functional channels, and they are used to control the external use of the vitalities forces, for health and spiritual purposes. If you can get this far, then you are on your way to spiritual immortality through Taoist alchemy.

**Yin/Yang**
This is a series of breathing exercises whereby the in-breath is as strong and takes as long as the out-breath. This style of breathing attracts energy from both heaven and earth, in equal measure. (See Diagram 4.)

The Yin Micro-cosmic Orbit, Yin/Yang section, consists of raising the breath and internal energy from the lower abdomen to the solar plexus and then driving it downward back to the abdomen. Placing one's hands on those two spots aids the circling of the energy, and also helps to vibrate and pulsate the psychic centres that are there.

The Yang Macro-cosmic Circle, Yin/Yang section, consists of lifting the breath and the internal energy through three levels,

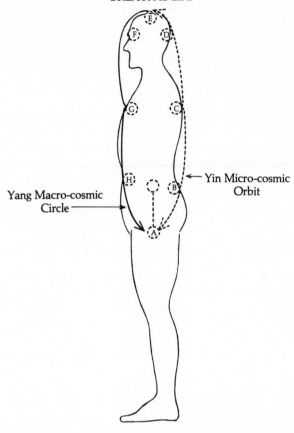

Diagram 3 Yang section: Yang Macro-cosmic Circle and Yin Micro-cosmic Orbit

from the lower stomach, into the solar plexus and then into the heart, and then gently lowering them back through the same centres until they rest again in their natural home, the lower abdomen.

In addition to the twenty basic breathing sequences in Taoism, there are many more, linked with physical movements and exercises. This makes the breathing and energy section of K'ai Men the most comprehensive and dynamic exploitation of the human body, the functions and vibrations of the psychic

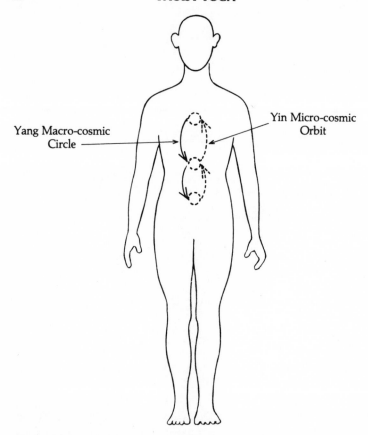

Diagram 4 Yin/Yang section: Yang Macro-cosmic Circle and Yin Micro-cosmic Orbit

centres, the contol channels to, from and within the mind, and the subconscious. The harmony of all opens the door to the spirit.

The importance of breathing is greatest at the beginning and end of your earthly life. Did you know that the first thing a baby does at birth is exhale, and that the last thing a dying person does is inhale? In the latter case, the pressure that has been built up by inhalation acts on the weakness of the heart and brings death.

All deep breathing brings about a harmony of Yin and Yang vibrations and pulsations, so learn to breathe deeply all the

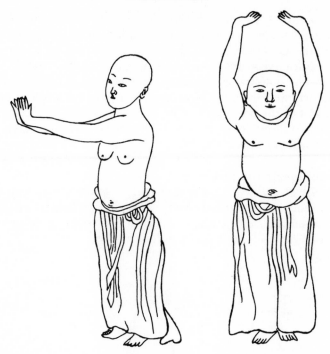

Diagram 5 Taoist "four-directional" Yang breathing exercise. Extracted from the *Book of Supple Muscles* (Ch'ing Period).

time, day in and day out, and utilize your full lung capacity, so that the body can obtain the maximum benefits. The various forms of healing in K'ai Men — meridian healing, Ch'i healing, breath healing, sound healing, meditation healing, Chinese push and pull massage, spot pressing and so on — are all founded upon the effective use of vibrations and pulsations.

In K'ai Men, great emphasis is placed on correct and total breathing — irrespective of the type of breathing exercise being executed — and upon maintaining complete breath control at all times. All physical exercises in K'ai Men are split into two sections: the "sequence", in which deep breathing is of particular importance; and the "extension", in which full and constant mind and body control are the speciality.

Regulated breathing under strictly controlled conditions will enable you to learn how to drive your breath downwards to the lower abdomen, so arousing the Lower Cauldron or Inner Fire, as it is sometimes known, and activating and pressurising the internal energy held there. This in turn activates that energy so that it is forced up and rises as you inhale. When you exhale this relaxes the diaphragm, which takes the pressure off the lower abdomen, and the internal energy then sinks back to it, down the front of the body.

There follow three different breathing exercises, each of which will in its own way help you internally.

**A Yang breath** (see Diagram 5)
This will give you a great deal of energy, and will warm up the whole body, so if you feel cold this is really excellent. It will also help to kill off the bacteria of the common cold and influenza, and will generally tone up the whole system.

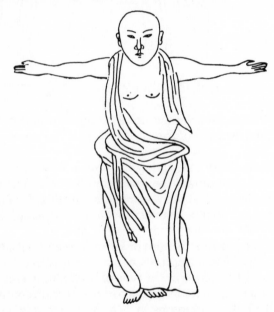

Stand with your feet about the width of your shoulders apart, and your hands by your sides.

1.   Breathe in through the nose and raise the hands in front of the shoulders as you do so. Exhale slowly but very forcibly

through the mouth, as you push slowly but strongly straight forward with the hands, extending the arms.

2. Breathe in through the nose and allow the hands to come back in front of the shoulders. Exhale slowly but very forcibly through the mouth, as you push slowly but strongly sideways with the hands, till the arms are fully extended.

3. Breathe in through the nose and allow the hands to come back in front of the shoulders. Exhale slowly but forcibly through the mouth, and as you do so push slowly but strongly directly upwards towards the ceiling.

4. Breathe in through the nose and allow the hands to come back in front of the shoulders. Exhale slowly but forcibly through the mouth and simultaneously push slowly but strongly downwards, till your arms are fully extended by your thighs.

Now repeat this sequence. You will really feel the benefits.

## A Yin breath

This breathing exercise is excellent to do at any time of day, and will help clear the nasal passages and soothe the nerves, and enable the body and mind to relax completely. If you ever feel tense, or under strain, or think a headache is coming on, then try this exercise.

You can sit down to do this exercise. Rest your right elbow on a table, and place the index finger of your right hand on your forehead, between your eyebrows (if you are left-handed, substitute left for right throughout the exercise).

1. Now press your right thumb against your right nostril so as to close that nostril completely. Slowly inhale through your left nostril until you have filled your chest as much as you can, and then exhale just as slowly through the same nostril until all the air has gone.

2. Now free your right nostril and press the middle finger of your right hand against your left nostril, so as to close it. Slowly breathe in again, filling your lungs and chest, and then slowly and completely exhale.

These two movements comprise the full sequence, and if you repeat it five times you will find it very relaxing indeed; but ensure that the breathing is done continuously and that there is no time lag in changing from thumb and middle finger or *vice versa*.

## A Yin/Yang breath

This exercise is excellent for the activation of energy and vibrates three psychic centres, which in turn revitalize the whole of the anatomy and mind.

Make yourself comfortable either by sitting in a chair or, better still, by sitting on the floor with your legs crossed. Keep the body upright, but do not hold it too stiffly. Place your right hand on your lower abdomen, and your left hand on the solar plexus — in both cases, directly on the skin.

1.   Now breathe in through the nose, but breathe deeply, so that the downward pressure pushes your right hand outward. Then press with your right hand on your lower abdomen so that the air is forced upward into the area of the solar plexus.
2.   Press with your left hand, so that the air is forced to rise up into the chest.
3.   Slowly exhale through the nose, allowing the chest to collapse.
4.   Press your left hand on the solar plexus so that all the air there is pushed out.
5.   Press with your right hand, so that all the air remaining in the lower abdomen is expelled.

Don't forget to breathe as deeply as you possibly can, and endeavour to do a minimum of six in- and out-breaths, following the above sequence.

Learn to breathe — and you will live.
Learn to breathe well — and you will retain good health.
Learn to breathe deep — and you will attain longevity.
Learn to breathe inwardly, without breathing —and you will gain spiritual immortality.
Follow the Taoist advice, now and always.

*Chapter 6*

# Hints for Good Practice

Everyone who is prepared to practise hard and diligently, and who has the mind to aim for the highest level, needs a helping hand and a few guidelines to help him along the way. The stresses and strains of work and home life, bringing up families, and the burdens that we all carry each day slowly sap our energy, and cause the body to run down, so that we do not always feel that we have the energy to carry on. Anger, jealousy, depression, worry and other emotions may put the mind under constant stress, making it very difficult to concentrate and think clearly.

To avoid this, the emotions must be brought under control, so that your response to events and to others remains on a constant level. This is hard to achieve, but once you have the strength of mind to get yourself under control every minute of every day, you will find life takes on a new dimension and a completely different aspect. There will be such peace, harmony and happiness within you that you may think a miracle has happened. But miracles don't happen, for it is the natural flow of nature and should be an every day occurrence, and we should learn to accept it as such, for this is the Tao.

**Sleep**
No one should ever sleep too much, because this can make the body become earthbound, and feel very heavy and sluggish. Anyone who is really healthy, especially someone who for at

least three years has cultivated Ch'ang Ming eating and drinking habits, needs only five to six hours sleep every night, irrespective of the type of work he does.

Make sure that you always sleep with the window open, so that there is always fresh air available in your bedroom. To avoid draughts, have only one window open at a time, and keep the door closed.

Do not have a bed too soft. A firm bed is much better for comfort and will help you to sleep more relaxed. If the bed sags, your body can be caused unnecessary strain, even though you are trying to relax. There is an old saying that "One hour's sleep before midnight is worth two hours' afterwards", and this is absolutely true. This is because after midnight the heart, small intestine, bladder, and kidneys are at their lowest ebb, the body temperature drops, breathing slows, and these organs work more slowly, so that they too can rest. As you can see from the following diagram which depicts the Yin and Yang aspects of a normal day, the early hours of the morning is also a Yin period:

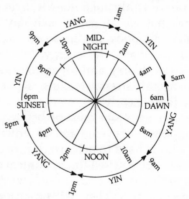

If you dream or have nightmares, or if you awaken during the night, then it is very likely that you will find that it is between 1 a.m. and 5 a.m.; so, it is vital to get as much sleep as possible before 1 a.m. for good health and complete relaxation and thereby ensuring that your body gets the maximum benefit from the rest.

**Vitality**
In China it has been known for thousands of years that the

organs, blood, mind, spirit, body, our psychic spheres, and our energies, indeed, all living things in the universe move through regular cycles of minimum and maximum activity. The annual cycle is as follows:

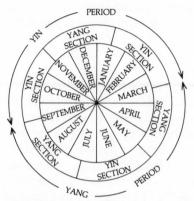

So everyone is at their lowest ebb in December, and at maximum vitality in June, but individuals vary slightly depending on when they were born, but such variation will not exceed three weeks. There are also monthly and daily vitality cycles.

The following diagram shows the times of the day at which the principal organs of the body are at their peak condition. These times are calculated with reference to the "lines of meridian" of the human body, and which are used in most

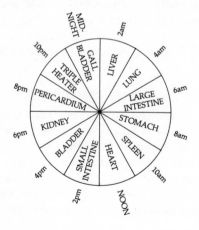

Chinese healing arts such as the Eight Strands of the Brocade, which includes spot pressing, vibration healing, Ch'i healing, Li healing, push and pull massage, sound healing, as well as being used extensively in acupuncture.

So if you have heart trouble get to bed before 11 p.m., and if you have lung trouble don't do anything really active between 3 and 5 p.m.

## Relaxation
If you live the Ch'ang Ming way you will not feel tired or fatigued, and thus will be unlikely to fall ill, for tiredness is one of the basic causes of illness. However, if you feel at all tense at anytime, sit quietly, with your back upright (do *not* slump down in an armchair!), and relax your mind and your whole body. Close your eyes if this helps, and try to erase the sounds that come into your ears and mind. Try a few deep breathing exercises, such as the "Yin breath", described in Chapter 5. This will help you to relax and at the same time will increase the oxygen in your bloodstream.

Tensions can also be reduced by taking a shower or bath before practising K'ai Men, and you will benefit too by taking one afterwards. If your eyes are heavy or you have a slight head-ache, lie on the floor, with your tongue in the roof of the mouth, and breathe deeply through the lower abdomen (Tan T'ien). At the same time place your right hand on your eyes between your two eyebrows, making sure that the palm of your hand is in complete contact with your skin and eyelids, and with your left hand gently press on the floor with your fingertips, in a rhythm very similar to your own pulse. Do this for about one minute and you will be surprised how wonderful you feel afterwards.

## Food
The advantages of eating the Ch'ang Ming way have already been emphasized (see Chapter 4). Try it for six months, and you will be surprised how fit and alive you feel, how well you look, and in what good condition your skin is.

However, it is advisable never to eat just before practice, and after a very heavy meal you must allow at least three to four hours to go by before you attempt the exercises of K'ai Men. When you do eat, always chew each mouthful fifty to a hundred times, so that it turns to water before swallowing. This will ensure that you do not overload the stomach and that you never suffer from indigestion and ulcers.

## Time and Place of Practice
You can practise anywhere at any time of the day, but the ideal times are one hour after sunrise and one hour before sunset. Because of work commitments, however, you may find it best to practise in the evenings; but do try to practise at a regular time. K'ai Men exercises are such that you can do just a few at a time, so a practice session need last no longer than fifteen to twenty minutes.

Whenever you practise, make sure that the room in which you do so is clean and airy, without any draughts, and that the atmosphere is not cold or damp. You can even practise on bare floorboards, providing that the floor is even, so that when you lie on your back your spinal column is not rubbing against a knot in the woodwork. The ideal place to practise is on a carpet in a room with one window open.

## Clothing
This should be loose, so that you can bend and turn your body without the slightest restriction. The best clothing to wear for K'ai Men practice was developed in China over 5,000 years ago, and is ideal for all callisthenics, no matter how strenuous the movements may be.

## Breathing
This has already been covered in detail in Chapter 5. Suffice it to say here that deep breathing is essential.

In addition, learn to savour the golden nectar of your own body by keeping your tongue in the roof of your mouth all the time. As your mouth fills up with saliva, gently lift the chin, and swallow smoothly at one go. Get in the habit of doing this and you will be surprised at how beneficial it is.

## Mind
In everything that you try to do, concentrate fully at all times and learn to feel everything that goes on inside your own body. Learn also to concentrate on things and people around you.

Through concentration, and attention to even the smallest thing that happens, you will eventually learn to see the Tao all around you constantly, and you will begin to see and appreciate the path of your life.

This concentration will not only help you to strengthen your mind, and improve your memory, but also give you a very peaceful and tranquil outlook, because concentration will stop you worrying unnecessarily about incidentals.

The mental processes affect the emotions, and thus conscious control of the mind and its thoughts will induce a feeling of calmness, to the benefit of your mental and physical health and even of your subconscious mind, which will thereby become more relaxed. This in turn will see that you dream less and sleep more deeply. Concentration of your mental faculties will not only give you added inner power, but also give you an inner peace, which you may find remarkable.

In addition to all this, you will find your memory will get better and better, which it should do, for memory is based on experience in time, and as you get older your experience is greater, and therefore your memory should increase with your years.

### Bowels

Ensure that you empty the bowels and the bladder before you start your K'ai Men practice, because inner cleanliness is absolutely vital to your good health, and if you retain such waste matter within your system you may find that when you practise some of the exercises you feel restricted, which in turn could create a certain amount of tension. In addition, the effect of having waste matter in the body for long periods will be to reduce the purity of the blood, causing headaches and sluggishness.

Make sure that you go to the toilet regularly and try to cultivate a habit of going first thing each morning. This will clear the toxic matters that have accumulated in the body during the period you have been asleep.

### Menstruation

During menstruation it is best not to practise exercises in which the legs have to be in the air, or in which the body is bent forwards. Exercises in which the body is kept upright are best at such times.

## Menopause

For most women the menopause is a difficult time, marked by nervousness and periods of depression. Ch'ang Ming and dedicated practice of K'ai Men are the best answers, since they keep the body healthy and the mind calm and relaxed, so that the change is scarcely apparent and is easily accepted.

## Exercising

K'ai Men can be practised by anyone who will take the very little trouble required to do so. We suggest that, if you are a beginner and have never done physical exercises before, for the first month of practice you should keep to just the sequences of each exercise, practising regularly every day. The body will then become soft and relaxed, and you will be able to progress to the extensions of the exercises.

## Happiness

The man of the Tao is free from anger, hate, fear, and worry at all times, and if you live the Ch'ang Ming way as well then illness and suffering will not exist for you. You will be happy and pleasant all the time, and your appearance, your behaviour and your manners will radiate this happiness, pleasure, and relaxed air that you will have about you all the time. It will catch on, and others may ask you for the secret. When you tell them that it is no secret, but the natural way of life, and that you now recognize your predestined path, they will either want to join you in this knowledge, or secretly laugh behind your back. If they want to laugh, let them, for they are the ones losing out, not you, for you have attained an understanding of life and of nature, and of the universe that will be the envy of everyone. Do, however, try to pass on your understanding to others, so that all may benefit by the wonderful work of the Supreme Spirit.

We exist in this world with many, so let us try to help many on the way.

## Chapter 7

# Postures

The Chinese, Indian and Western styles of physical exercising are all vastly different from each other. The Western style concentrates on developing powerful muscles, generally with the help of mechanical aids, and thus the exercises are often hard and aggressive. The Indian style is much lighter in practise, but still tends to produce strong muscles, but it is less strenuous and is aimed at producing suppleness and dexterity as well. The Chinese style, however, concentrates entirely on developing the flexibility, adaptability and suppleness of the body as a whole. This it does through a form of internal massage known as "movement with stillness" (Yun Tung Pu Yun Tung) or, literally translated, "movement with no movement". The dynamic effects of this type of exercising are acknowledged by all who have practised it.

For thousands of years the number of basic postures or stances (Tzu Shih) were eight, and so it remained until Bodhidharma came from India and joined the Shaolin Temple. He increased the number of stances to eighteen, which even by modern standards were very hard, strenuous and toughening. All these stances had to be held for long periods at a time, and were intended to make the mind strong and dedicated, using discipline and emotional control to overcome physical pain and discomfort. Most of the Chinese monks who studied and practised under the direction of Bodhidharma found that the new discipline was far too hard and rigid and thus clashed physically, spiritually and mentally with the ancient Chinese ideas of internal development (Nei Kung), on which their training had originally been based. Thus, while many stuck at this unrelenting discipline for many years, a lot did not.

Since those early days K'ai Men has developed a great deal, the mental application becoming softer and more gentle over the centuries. The number of basic postures has increased to forty-two, but unfortunately it is not possible to incorporate all of them in this one volume, as the number of exercises involved is over 400. In addition to these basic postures and exercises, there are also advanced postures and the exercises that go with them, for teachers and the most advanced pupils.

We recommend that everyone, irrespective of age, learns to move from one posture to another, for this will help the body to loosen, relax and warm up before serious training commences. It will also aid the concentration of the mind, which is the first step to complete self-control.

### Double Plough Stance
### *(Shuang Chang Li Shih)*

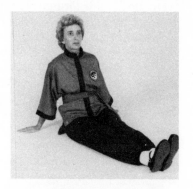

Sit on the floor with both legs stretched out in front of the body. The hands should rest on the floor slightly to the rear of the hips.

### Single Plough Stance
### *(Tan Chang Li Shih)*

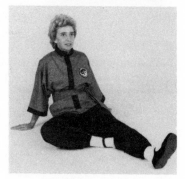

From the Double Plough Stance move one leg over the top of the other (or move it away to the side), leaving one leg stretched out in front.

### Lotus Leaf Stance
*(Ho Hua Yeh Shih)*

From the Double Plough Stance, bend both knees and draw the feet in. Then lower the knees outward toward the floor and move the soles of the feet together, so that they touch.

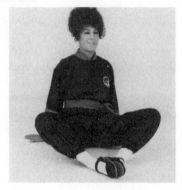

### Drunkard Stance
*(Tsui Han Shih)*

From the Double Plough Stance bring your hands to your sides, and lie back on to the floor.

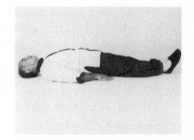

### Willow Tree Stance
*(Liu Shu Shih)*

From the Drunkard Stance, raise both legs into the air, so that they are perpendicular. (An advanced version of this is to raise the body and legs into the air, supporting the body on the hands and arms).

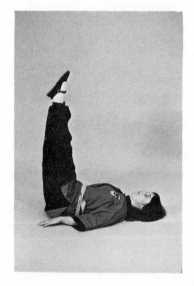

### Fish Stance
### *(Yu Shih)*

From the Drunkard Stance turn onto your right side and support your head with your right hand and arm. Then roll over onto your left side, and support your head with your left hand and arm.

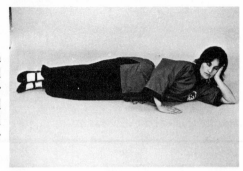

### Cobra Stance
### *(Yenching Shih)*

From the Drunkard Stance, roll over onto your front, and place your forearms on the floor close to your body, with your hands in front of your shoulders.

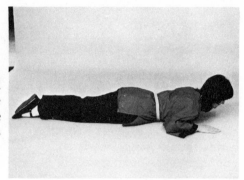

### Praying Mantis Stance
### *(Tao Lang Shih)*

From the Cobra Stance, push yourself up so that you are sitting on your own heels, and place your hands on your thighs.

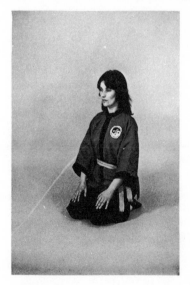

### Turtle Stance
*(Pie Shih)*

From the Praying Mantis Stance, place your hands on the floor about sixteen inches in front of your knees, and distribute the weight of your body evenly on your hands and knees.

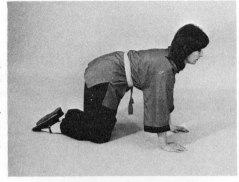

### Eagle Stance
*(Tiao Shih)*

From the Turtle Stance push yourself up onto your feet and bring your feet together. Your hands should hang loosely by your hips, eyes looking straight ahead.

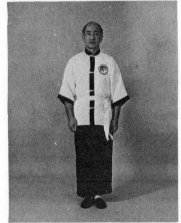

### Bear Stance
*(Hsiung Shih)*

From the Eagle Stance step sideways with your left foot so that your feet are about the width of your shoulders apart. Then move back to Eagle Stance and step the same distance to the right.

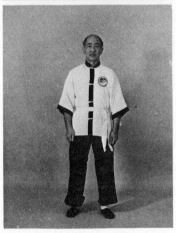

### Leg Triangle Stance
*(T'ui Sanchiao Shih)*

From the Bear Stance bend forward and put your left hand or the fingertips of your left hand on the floor just in front of your right foot. Then do likewise with the other hand and foot.

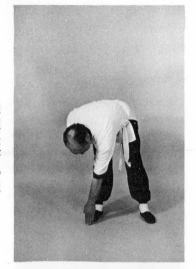

### Dragon Stance
*(Lung Shih)*

From the Eagle or Bear Stance step forward with your right leg so that your right foot is about a pace and a half in front of your other foot, and place most of your weight on your right leg. Return to your starting position and do likewise with your left foot and leg.

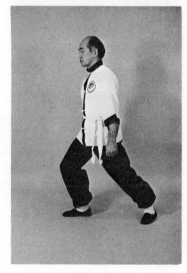

## Monkey Stance
### (Hou Shih)

From the Dragon Stance transfer your body weight fully onto
the rear leg, and allow the front
foot to slide back, till the feet
are about twelve inches apart.

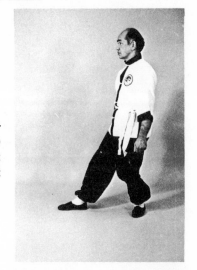

## Leopard Stance
### (Pao Shih)

From the Bear Stance place
your body weight on your left
leg and lean slightly to the right.
Then transfer your weight to
your right leg and lean to the
left.

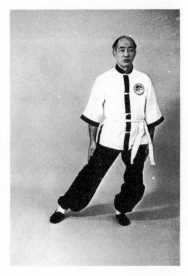

### Riding Horse Stance
*(Ch'i Ma Shih)*

From the Bear Stance step sideways so that your feet are more than the width of your shoulders apart. Bend both knees and distribute your body weight evenly on both legs.

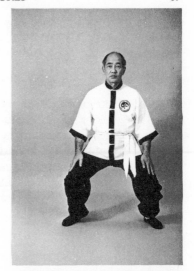

### Chicken Stance
*(Hsiao Chi Shih)*

From the Riding Horse Stance turn to the left and place most of your weight on your left leg. Bend the right leg so that your right knee is about an inch from the floor.

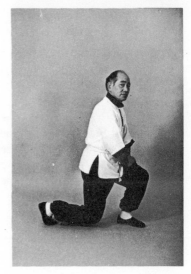

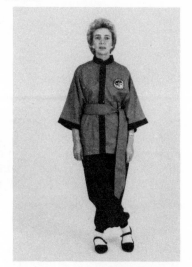

### Crossed-Leg Stance
*(Ch'iao-Cho T'su Shih)*

From the Bear or Eagle stance place the weight of the body onto one leg. Then move the other leg in front of and beyond the leg that is supporting your weight. The toes of the foot that is moved in front should rest lightly on the floor.

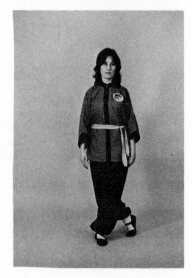

### Scissor Stance
*(Chien Tao Shih)*

This is the reverse of the Crossed-Leg Stance. While one leg supports your weight the other leg is moved behind and round it, till the toes rest on the floor.

## Chapter 8

# Movement with Stillness

For the benefit of anyone wishing to attempt the exercises described in this chapter, here are a few hints and pointers.

1. All exercises are split into two sections: the sequence and the extension. *Never* try the extension before you have run through the sequence.
2. For the first year, go through the sequence twice before going on to the extension; then go through the extension twice.
3. All exercises should be practised very slowly and evenly throughout.
4. Carry out all movements smoothly and gently, without sudden starts and changes.
5. The body goes through Yin and Yang phases, and this affects your performance. Do not, therefore, compare your performance on one day with that on another.
6. Do as much practice as you feel capable of doing, but never try to do more — even though you may feel that you have done better in the past.
7. *Never* hold any movement in the extensions. As soon as you reach your peak, immediately give way.
8. Concentrate on the muscle change that takes place, and try and feel where and how each one takes place within yourself.
9. Enjoy the glow of vitality that surges through you when you practise K'ai Men exercises.

*Exercise 1    Single Plough Stance (Tan Chang Li Shih)*

*Starting Position*
Sit on the floor with both legs stretched out in front, and rest both hands on the floor, just slightly to the rear of the hips. Rest your body weight on them and relax completely within yourself.

*Sequence movements*
1. BREATHE IN — as you cross your left leg over your right leg, bending the left knee so that your left ankle rests just above your right knee.
2. BREATHE OUT — as you grip your left ankle with your left hand, and your left foot with your right hand.
3. BREATHE IN — as you slowly rotate your left foot in a half circle, forward and down, using your right hand to accomplish the motion.
4. BREATHE OUT — as you complete the full circle of your left foot with your right hand.
5-6-7-8. Repeat Sequence Movements 3 and 4 twice more as you breathe in and out with every half circle of your left foot.
9. BREATHE IN — as you take your hands back on to the floor slightly to the rear of your hips, and relax your body.
10. BREATHE OUT — as you uncross your left leg, straighten it, and place it back on the floor alongside your right leg.
Repeat the above sequence, changing "left" for "right" and *vice versa.*

*Extension movements*
You should adopt your normal breathing when executing all Extension Movements.
1. As Sequence Movement 1.
2. As Sequence Movement 2, but as you grip your left foot fit the heel of your right thumb under the base of your big toe, with your fingers gripping round the little toe edge of your foot. Now turn your foot outward, so that the sole of the foot faces the ceiling, and keeping it in that position start the next movement.
3. As Sequence Movement 3, but executed very, very slowly.

4. As Sequence Movement 4, but again very slowly.
5-6-7-8. Repeat 3 and 4.
9. As Sequence Movement 9.
10. As Sequence Movement 10.
Repeat the Extension Movements, changing "left" for "right" and *vice versa*.

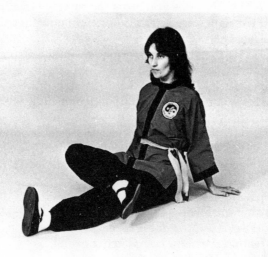

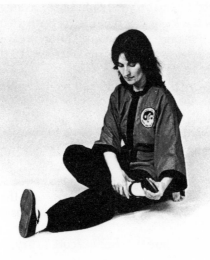

*Exercise 2     Single Plough Stance (Tan Chang Li Shih)*

*Starting position*
This is the same as Exercise 1.

*Sequence movements*
1. BREATHE IN — as you cross the right leg over the left leg.
   Bend the right knee so that your right ankle rests just above
   your left knee.
2. BREATHE OUT — as you grip your right foot with your left
   hand and draw your right foot towards your left hip.
3. BREATHE IN — and allow your right foot to slide back
   towards your left knee, by gently pushing with your left
   hand.
4. BREATHE OUT — as you raise and straighten your right leg,
   and place it alongside your left leg on the floor.
Repeat the above sequence, changing "right" to "left" and *vice
versa*.

*Extension movements*
During the execution of these Extension Movements ensure that
your breathing remains completely normal.
1. As Sequence Movement 1.
2. As Sequence Movement 2.
3. Place your right hand on your right knee, and gently and very
   slowly press the knee downwards towards the floor. When
   you reach the stage when you cannot press it down any
   further, then release pressure immediately and allow the knee
   to rise slowly to its natural position.
4. Push gently with the left hand to allow the right ankle to slide
   back towards the left knee.
5. Raise and straighten your right leg, and place it back on the
   floor alongside your left leg.
Repeat the extension, changing "right" for "left" and *vice versa*.

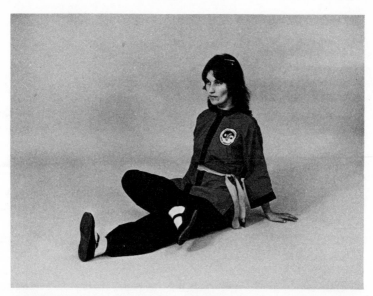

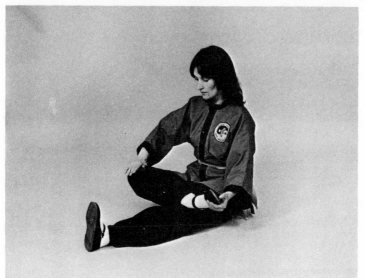

*Exercise 3    Single Plough Stance (Tan Chang Li Shih)*

*Starting position*
This is the same as Exercise 1.

*Sequence movements*
1. BREATHE IN — as you draw your right foot up to the outside of your right thigh, and drop the right knee to the floor.
2. BREATHE OUT — and raise the right knee and slide your right foot back to the starting position.
3. BREATHE IN — and simultaneously draw your left foot up to the outside of your left thigh, and drop the left knee on to the floor.
4. BREATHE OUT — as you raise your left knee and allow your left foot to slide back to the starting position.
5. BREATHE IN — and draw up both feet as far as possible so that the right foot is outside the right thigh, and left foot outside the left thigh, and lower both knees downwards towards the floor.
6. BREATHE OUT — raising both knees, and sliding both feet back to the starting position.
Repeat the above sequence once more.

*Extension movements*
Let your breathing be completely normal during these Extension Movements.
1. As Sequence Movement 1.
2. As Sequence Movement 2, but make sure that as you slide your right foot back to the starting position you keep your right knee in contact with the floor all the time.
3. As Sequence Movement 3.
4. As Sequence Movement 4, but ensure that as you slide your left foot back to the starting position you keep your left knee on the floor all the time.
5. As Sequence Movement 5.
6. As Sequence Movement 6, but endeavour to keep both knees as low as you can, on the floor if possible, while you slide both feet back to the starting position.
Repeat all the Extension Movements once more.

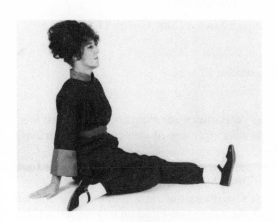

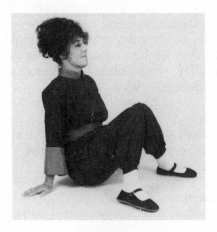

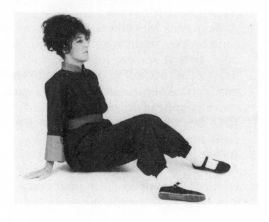

*Exercise 4    Single Plough Stance (Tan Chang Li Shih)*

*Starting position*
Exactly the same as Exercise 1.

*Sequence movements*
1. BREATHE IN — as you draw your right foot back till it is at least on a level with your right hip (if you can take it further, so much the better).
2. BREATHE OUT — as you touch the sole of your right foot with the palm of your right hand.
3. BREATHE IN — as you take your right hand off the sole of your right foot, and place the same hand on to your left ankle.
4. BREATHE OUT — as you take your right hand and right leg back to the starting position.
5. BREATHE IN — whilst drawing your left foot back till it is on a level with your left hip, or further if you can.
6. BREATHE OUT — whilst touching the sole of your left foot with the palm of your left hand.
7. BREATHE IN — as you now place your left hand on the ankle of your right leg.
8. BREATHE OUT — as you now take your left hand and left leg back to their original starting positions.
Repeat the above sequence once again.

*Extension movements*
Breathing should be completely normal during the extension movements.
1. As Sequence Movement 1.
2. As Sequence Movement 2, but once having put your right hand on your right sole, then slowly turn your body to the right, so that you can look over your right shoulder.
3. Release the touch of your right palm on the sole of your right foot, and take both hands down to your left ankle, grip it, and lower your head downwards towards your left knee.
4. Take both hands and your right leg back to the starting position.
5. As Sequence Movement 5.
6. As Sequence Movement 6, but having put your left hand on your left sole, slowly turn your body round to the left, and look over your left shoulder.

7. Take your left hand off the sole of your left foot, and take both hands down so that you can grip your right ankle. Having done so then lower your head down towards your right knee.
8. Release your grips and take both hands and your left leg back to the starting position.
Repeat the above eight numbers once more.

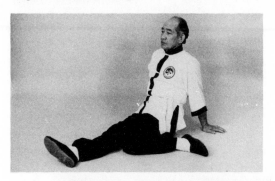

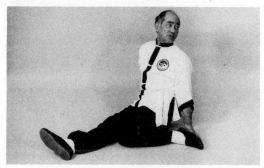

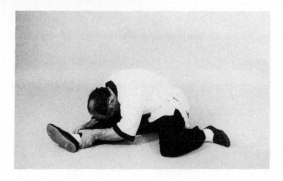

*Exercise 5    Double Plough Stance (Shuang Chang Li Shih)*

*Starting position*
The same as Exercise 1.

*Sequence movements*
1. BREATHE IN — as you draw your right foot in until the sole
   is near the inside of your left knee.
2. BREATHE OUT — as you then move your right foot
   outwards and inwards in a big circle round to the starting
   position.
3. BREATHE IN — drawing your left foot inwards till the sole is
   near to the inside of your right knee.
4. BREATHE OUT — circling the left foot outwards and
   inwards back to the starting position.
5. BREATHE IN — whilst drawing in both feet, until the soles
   touch one another.
6. BREATHE OUT — and separate the feet and circle them
   outwards and then inwards until they are both back to the
   starting position.
Repeat the full sequence once more.

*Extension movements*
Remember to breathe normally.
1. As Sequence Movement 1.
2. As Sequence Movement 2, but keep the outside edge of your
   right foot in contact with the floor as long as you can, till it is
   back at the starting position.
3. As Sequence Movement 3.
4. As Sequence Movement 4, but try and keep the outside edge
   of your left foot in constant contact with the floor, until it is
   back in the original starting position.
5. As Sequence Movement 5.
6. As Sequence Movement 6, but try to keep the outside edge of
   both feet in contact with the floor as long as you can, till they
   are both back at the starting position.
Repeat these six Extension Movements again.

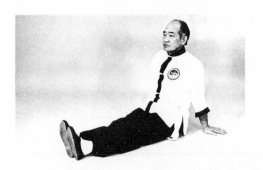

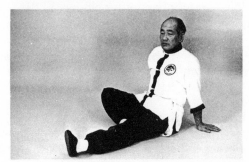

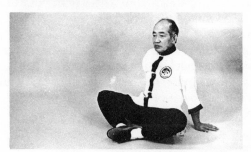

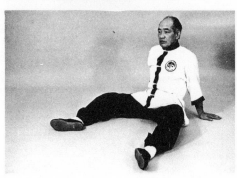

*Exercise 6    Double Plough Stance (Shuang Chang Li Shih)*

*Starting position*
The same as Exercise 1.

*Sequence movements*
1. BREATHE IN — bending slightly forward and putting your hands on the calves of your legs.
2. BREATHE OUT — as you straighten your body and put your hands on the floor behind your hips.
3. BREATHE IN — as you bend your elbows a little, and lean slightly backwards.
4. BREATHE OUT — as you straighten your arms and your body to the original starting position — now relax.
Repeat the above four movements.

*Extension movements*
Remember to breathe quite normally.
1. Bend deeply forward as you grip the calves of your legs, and allow your elbows to bend as much as they can, whilst you endeavour to touch your knees with your head.
2. As Sequence Movement 2.
3. Lean backwards as far as you can, allowing your elbows to bend as deeply as possible, and at the same time let your head move as far back as it can.
4. Straighten your arms, head and your body until you assume the starting position. Now relax completely.
Repeat these four extensions once more.

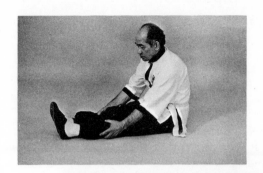

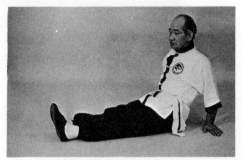

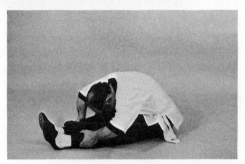

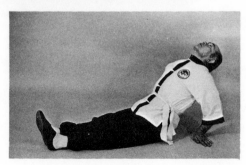

## Exercise 7    Double Plough Stance (Shuang Chang Li Shih)

*Starting position*
The same as Exercise 1.

*Sequence movements*
1. BREATHE IN — as you lean back so that your body weight rests on your hands, and at the same time raise the body upwards until it is in a straight line from head to feet.
2. BREATHE OUT — as you lower your body back to the floor and return to the starting position.
3. BREATHE IN — as you bend forward until you can touch your toes with the tips of your fingers of both hands.
4. BREATHE OUT — as you return to the starting position.
Repeat the above sequences once more.

*Extension movements*
Breathing should be normal whilst executing the extensions.
1. As Sequence Movement 1, but as you raise your body into the air, push your tummy upwards towards the ceiling, and at the same time slowly take your head backwards as far as you can.
2. As Sequence Movement 2.
3. As Sequence Movement 3, but very slowly stretch your fingers beyond your toes, and at the same time take your head down as low as you can.
4. As Sequence Movement 4.
Repeat these Extension Movements once again.

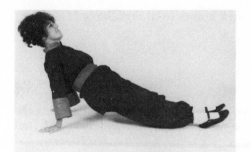

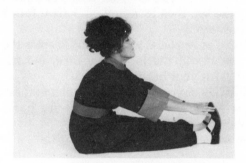

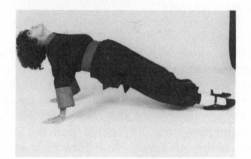

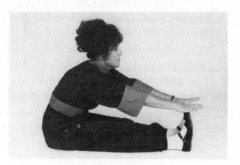

*Exercise 8    Double Plough Stance (Shuang Chang Li Shih)*

*Starting position*
The same as Exercise 1.

*Sequence movements*
1. BREATHE IN — as you bend your right leg, and keeping the sole of the right foot on the floor, draw your right heel towards your buttocks.
2. BREATHE OUT — as you lift your right foot into the air, straightening the leg, then lowering your right foot back to the starting position.
3. BREATHE IN — as you bend your left leg, keeping the sole of that foot in contact with the floor all the time, and draw your left heel in towards your buttocks.
4. BREATHE OUT — as you lift your left foot into the air, then straighten the leg, then lower the whole leg back to the starting position.
Repeat the four Sequence Movements once again.

*Extension movements*
Keep breathing normally whilst executing the extension movements.
1. As in Sequence Movement 1, then grip your ankle with both hands and draw your right heel as close to your buttocks as you can, then lower your head to the left (or inside) of your right knee. Taking your head down as far as possible.
2. Straighten your body and raise your right leg into the air, straightening it out, by locking the knee, and grip your right ankle with both hands. Now draw your ankle towards your head, but keep your head upright.
3. Release your grips on the ankle and place both hands back on the floor to the rear of your hips, and at the same time lower your right leg back to the floor to the original starting position.
4. The same as Extension 1, but substitute "left" for "right".
5. The same as Extension 2, but substitute "left" for "right".
6. The same as Extension 3, but substitute "left" for "right".
Repeat these six Extension Movements once more.

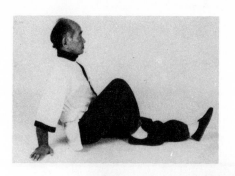

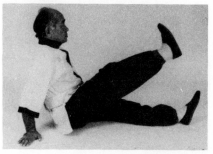

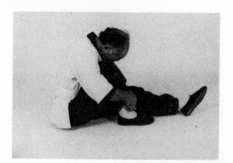

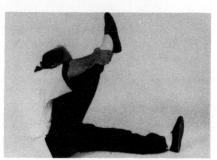

*Exercise 9    Double Plough Stance (Shuang Chang Li Shih)*

*Starting position*
The same as Exercise 1.

*Sequence movements*
1. BREATHE IN — as you place your hands on your lap.
2. BREATHE OUT — as you turn your body to the right, and place both hands on the floor by the hips and thighs.
3. BREATHE IN — as you turn back to the front, placing both hands on your lap.
4. BREATHE OUT — as you turn your body to the left, placing both hands on the floor by your hips and thighs.
5. BREATHE IN — as you turn back to the front, placing both hands on your lap.
6. BREATHE OUT — as you take your hands back on to the floor behind your hips and relax in the starting position.
Repeat the above Sequence Movements once again.

*Extension movements*
Remember, when executing the extensions, breathing should be normal.
1. As Sequence Movement 1.
2. Turn your body to the right, and place both hands on the floor by the hips and thighs. Now very slowly turn your body round to the right as far as it will go, and at the same time push your right hand strongly on the floor to help your turn. The head also turns to the right as you try and look over your right shoulder.
3. As Sequence Movement 3.
4. Turn your body to the left, placing both hands on the floor by your hips and thighs. As you push firmly on the floor with your left hand, slowly turn your body and head round to the left as far as you can go, and at the same time see if you can look over your left shoulder.
5. As Sequence Movement 5.
6. As Sequence Movement 6.
Repeat the extensions once more, on both sides of the body.

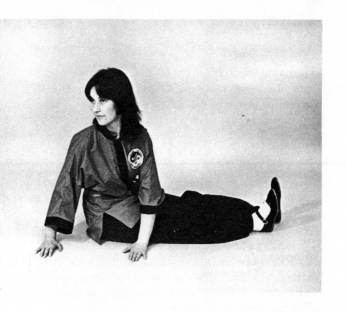

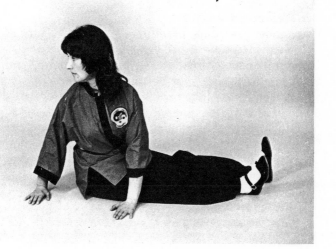

*Exercise 10   Lotus Leaf Stance (Ho Hua Yeh Shih)*

*Starting position*
The same as Exercise 1.

*Sequence movements*
1. BREATHE IN — as you bend your knees, and grip the ankles, then pull the legs inwards so that your heels come close to your buttocks, and the soles of both feet are together.
2. BREATHE OUT — as you lean slightly forward with the body, and at the same time tilt the head slightly back.
3. BREATHE IN — as you straighten the head and body.
4. BREATHE OUT — as you lean the body slightly backwards, and simultaneously allow the head to droop forward so your chin is nearly touching your chest.
5. BREATHE IN — as you straighten your body and head.
6. BREATHE OUT — as you straighten your legs and take your hands back to the rear of your hips, so that you are once more in the starting posture.
Repeat the complete sequence of six movements once more.

*Extension movements*
Reminder — that breathing is normal during extension movements.
1. As Sequence Movement 1, but this time try and pull your heels as close to your bottom as you can.
2. As Sequence Movement 2, but lean as far forward as you can, and at the same time tilt your head back as far as possible.
3. As Sequence Movement 3.
4. As Sequence Movement 4, but lean back to your maximum and as you bend your head forward try and press your chin into your chest.
5. As Sequence Movement 5.
6. As Sequence Movement 6.
Repeat the above six Extension Movements.

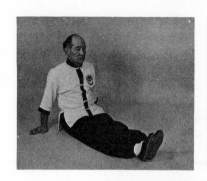 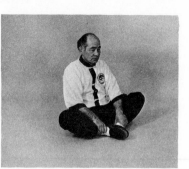

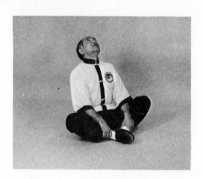

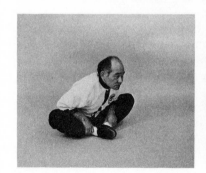 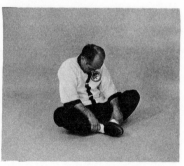

*Exercise 11    Lotus Leaf Stance (Ho Hua Yeh Shih)*

*Starting position*
As in Exercise 1.

*Sequence movements*
1. BREATHE IN — as you bend your knees, grip your ankles, and draw the feet towards your buttocks, keeping the soles of the feet together.
2. BREATHE OUT — as you release the grip on your ankles, and move both legs outwards in a big circle, and then inwards, eventually straightening them so that they resume the starting position. Your hands meanwhile should go back naturally on to the floor to the rear of your hips, as soon as you release the grip on your ankles.
Now repeat the above sequences twice more.

*Extension movements*
Breathing remains normal during the following movements.
1. As Sequence Movement 1, but endeavour to pull your feet in as far as you possibly can.
2. Transfer your hands from the ankles to a point under the little toes of your feet. Now with both hands lift the toes of both feet, but still keep the heels in contact with the floor.
3. Hold the toes in the extended position with your right hand, whilst your left hand is used to press on your left knee in a downwards direction towards the floor.
4. Now change hands, with the left hand holding the toes in the extension position, and your right hand pressing downwards on your right knee.
5. Release both hands and transfer them back to the position on the floor just to the rear of your hips, as in the starting position.
6. Now move your legs outwards in a big circle, then inwards towards one another, so that you are once more back in the starting position.
Repeat these Extension Movements once more.

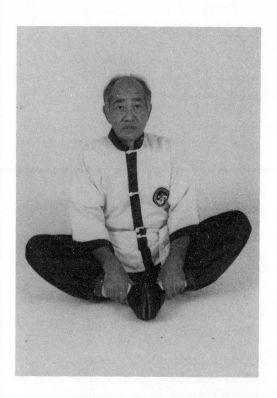

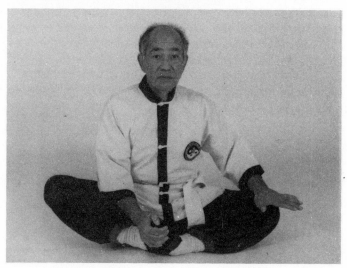

*Exercise 12    Turtle Stance (Pie Shih)*

*Starting position*
Kneel on the floor, sitting on the heels, with toes pointing to the
rear, and your body erect but relaxed.

*Sequence movements*
1. BREATHE IN — as you move your body forward so that
   your hands rest on the floor directly under your shoulders;
   with arms and thighs now being perpendicular. Keep the
   back straight, and the head facing straight down.
2. BREATHE OUT — as you arc your back into the air.
3. BREATHE IN — as you straighten your back.
4. BREATHE OUT — as you hollow or dip your back so that
   your abdomen is pushed downward.
5. BREATHE IN — as you raise your back so that it straightens
   out once more.
6. BREATHE OUT — as you take your hands off the floor, and
   sit back on your heels and relax.
Repeat the above sequence once more.

*Extension movements*
Your normal breathing is expected during these extensions.
1. As Sequence Movement 1.
2. As Sequence Movement 2, but try to raise your back as high
   as you possibly can into the air, and as you do so bend your
   head downwards and try and look between your own legs.
3. As Sequence Movement 3.
4. As Sequence Movement 4, but as you dip your back and push
   your abdomen downwards towards the floor, take your head
   as far back as you can.
5. As Sequence Movement 5.
6. As Sequence Movement 6.
Go through these Extension Movements once more.

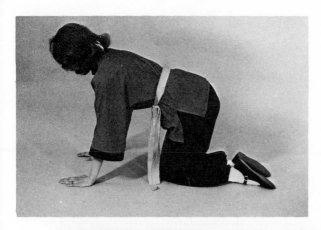

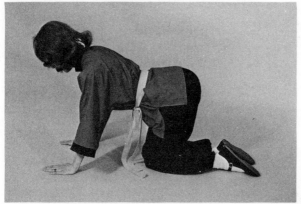

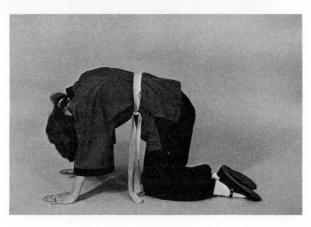

*Exercise 13    Turtle Stance (Pie Shih)*

*Starting position*
The same as in Exercise 12.

*Sequence movements*
1. BREATHE IN — as you bend forward and place both hands
   on the floor, with your back straight. The arms and thighs
   should be upright.
2. BREATHE OUT — as you let your body move forward,
   without moving the hands, so that your shoulders are slightly
   ahead of your wrists.
3. BREATHE IN — as you slowly move back until your
   shoulders are over the wrists, and the arms and thighs
   perpendicular.
4. BREATHE OUT — as you lift your buttocks into the air and
   straighten both legs.
5. BREATHE IN — as you lower your knees back on to the
   floor.
6. BREATHE OUT — as you take both hands off the floor, and
   sit back on to your heels, with your body upright. Now relax.
Repeat the complete sequence of six movements once more.

*Extension movements*
Breathing should be completely normal.
1. The same as Sequence Movement 1.
2. Same as Sequence Movement 2, but as your body moves
   forward try to look upwards by tilting the head backwards.
3. Same as Sequence Movement 3.
4. Same as Sequence Movement 4, but as you lift your buttocks
   into the air and straighten both legs, allow your head to bend
   forward and downwards and try and look through your legs.
5. As Sequence Movement 5, but as you lower your knees back
   to the floor, don't forget to straighten your head.
6. As Sequence Movement 6, returning to your starting
   position, and relax.
Repeat this set of Extension Movements again.

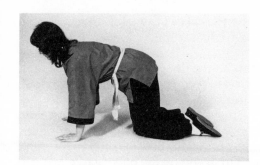

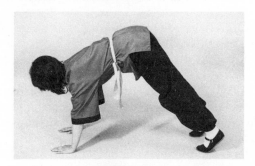

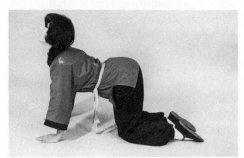

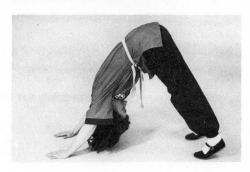

*Exercise 14    Praying Mantis Stance (Tao Lang Shih)*

*Starting position*
Sit in a kneeling position on the floor, buttocks on your heels and toes pointing to the rear. Your fingers should be resting on the floor alongside the feet.

*Sequence movements*
1. BREATHE IN — as you turn your body slightly to the right, and allow your left hand to rest on the outside of your right knee.
2. BREATHE OUT — as you raise your right arm sideways, to shoulder height.
3. BREATHE IN — as you lower your right arm back to the floor.
4. BREATHE OUT — as you turn back to the front and withdraw your left hand off your right knee and take your arm back to your left side, with the fingers touching the floor alongside your feet.
5. BREATHE IN — as you turn your body round to the left, and take your right hand forward so that it comes to rest on the outside of your left knee.
6. BREATHE OUT — as you raise your left arm sideways to shoulder height.
7. BREATHE IN — as you lower your left arm back to the floor.
8. BREATHE OUT — as you turn back to the front, taking your right hand off your left knee, and take your arm back to the starting position with your right fingers touching the floor alongside your right foot.
Now repeat this complete sequence of eight movements once more.

*Extension movements*
Normal breathing is sufficient during the following extensions.
1. As Sequence Movement 1.
2. As Sequence Movement 2, then drop your arm back behind your own back so you can grip your left side. Turn your head fully to the right.
3. Raise your right arm sideways, then lower it downwards so that your right fingers touch the floor as in the starting position.

4. As Sequence Movement 4.
5. As Sequence Movement 5.
6. Raise left arm sideways first, then drop it behind your own back so you can grip your right side. Head turned fully to the left.
7. Raise left arm sideways, then afterwards drop the whole arm downwards to the floor, so that your left fingers are by your left foot.
8. As Sequence Movement 8.
Repeat the Extension Movements once again.

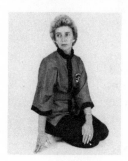

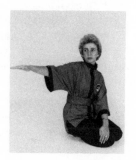

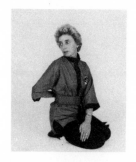

*Exercise 15     Praying Mantis Stance (Tao Lang Shih)*

*Starting position*
As in Exercise 14.

*Sequence movements*
1. BREATHE IN — as you lift your knees off the floor as you lean backwards slightly, pushing on your fingers.
2. BREATHE OUT — as you return to the starting position.
3. BREATHE IN — as you put your hands on the floor in front of your knees and bend the body forward.
4. BREATHE OUT — as you return to the starting position.
Repeat the sequence once more.

*Extension movements*
Keep your breathing completely normal.
1. As Sequence Movement 1, but lift your knees as high as you can and at the same time bend your body forward, trying to touch your knees with your chin.
2. As Sequence Movement 2.
3. Put your hands on the floor well in front of your knees so that arms and legs are perpendicular; then lift your feet as high as you can, and at the same time tilt your head as far back as you can.
4. Return to the starting position.
Repeat this extension once more.

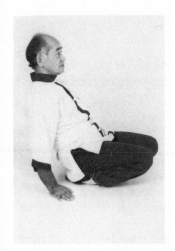

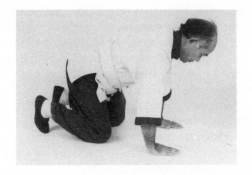

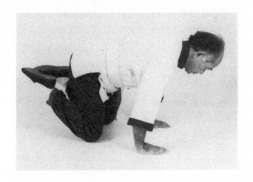

*Exercise 16    Drunkard Stance (Tsui Han Shih)*

*Starting position*
Lay flat on your back on the floor, hands by your sides with palms facing downwards, and your legs stretched out.

*Sequence movements*
1. BREATHE IN — as you raise your right leg in the air, simultaneously bending the knee.
2. BREATHE OUT — keeping your hands flat on the floor, turn your hips slightly to the left, and allow your right knee to move halfway towards the floor on your left side.
3. BREATHE IN — as you bring your right leg back to its position in Movement 1.
4. BREATHE OUT — as you straighten your body, and lower the leg back to the floor, so that you are once again in the starting position.
Repeat the sequence, changing "right" for "left" and *vice versa*.
Now repeat the complete sequence of eight movements, firstly four with the right leg, and then the four sequences with the left leg.

*Extension movements*
Keep your breathing normal during the following extensions.
1. As Sequence Movement 1.
2. As Sequence Movement 2, but this time as you turn your hips allow your right knee to drop to the floor by your left side.
3. As Sequence Movement 3.
4. As Sequence Movement 4.
Repeat the extension, changing "right" for "left" and *vice versa*.
Now repeat the eight movements once more, first with the right leg and then the left.

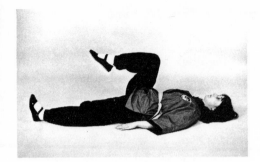

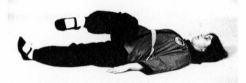

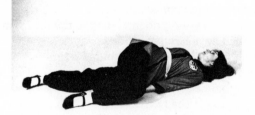

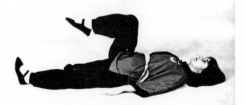

*Exercise 17    Drunkard Stance (Tsui Han Shih)*

*Starting position*
As in Exercise 16.

*Sequence movements*
1. BREATHE IN — as you lift your right leg into the air, bending the knee.
2. BREATHE OUT — straighten the leg so it is completely perpendicular.
3. BREATHE IN — as you bend the knee again.
4. BREATHE OUT — turning your hips slightly to the left, so that your right knee is about halfway to the floor.
5. BREATHE IN — straighten your leg again, and point your toes away.
6. BREATHE OUT — as you bend your knee once again.
7. BREATHE IN — as you straighten your body, and allow your right leg to move back to its natural position, with the thigh upright.
8. BREATHE OUT — as you lower your right leg back to the floor, straightening the leg as you do so, so that you return to the starting position.
Repeat the sequence again, using the left leg.

*Extension movements*
Retain your normal breathing pattern.
1. As Sequence Movement 1.
2. As Sequence Movement 2, but as the leg is straightened lift the head off the floor.
3. As Sequence Movement 3, but when you bend the leg, lower the head back to the floor.
4. As Sequence Movement 4, but lower the right knee so that it touches the floor to your left, and turn your head to the right so that you look over your right shoulder.
5. As Sequence Movement 5.
6. As Sequence Movement 6.
7. As Sequence Movement 7, but also straighten the head.
8. As Sequence Movement 8.

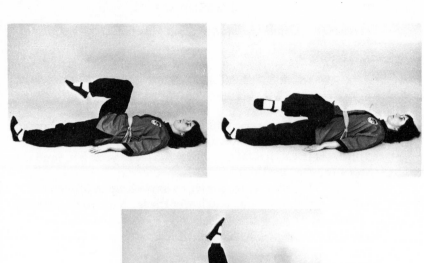

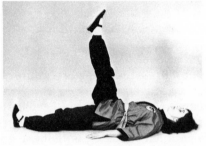

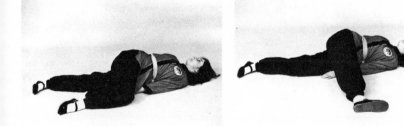

*Exercise 18  Drunkard Stance (Tsui Han Shih)*

*Starting position*
As in Exercise 16.

*Sequence movements*
1. BREATHE IN — raise your right leg straight up in the air, so that it ends up perpendicular with the toes pulled back.
2. BREATHE OUT — as you lower the leg to your left, until the foot touches the floor.
3. BREATHE IN — return the leg to its position in Movement 1.
4. BREATHE OUT — as you lower the leg back to the starting position.
Repeat the sequence, using the left leg.

*Extension movements*
Keep to your normal breathing procedure.
1. As Sequence Movement 1.
2. As Sequence Movement 2, but keeping the foot in contact with the floor all the time, slowly move the leg upwards towards your left shoulder, until it can go no further.
3. As Sequence Movement 3.
4. As Sequence Movement 4.
Repeat these Extension Movements using the left leg.

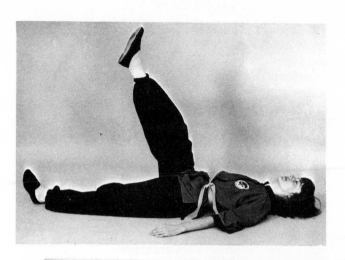

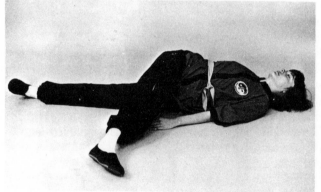

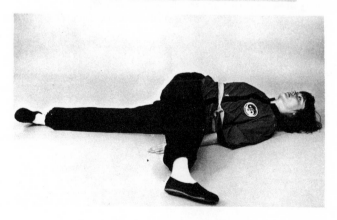

*Exercise 19　Drunkard Stance (Tsui Han Shih)*

*Starting position*
As in Exercise 16.

*Sequence movements*
1. BREATHE IN — as you raise your feet until they are about twelve inches from the floor.
2. BREATHE OUT — lifting your legs until they are perpendicular.
3. BREATHE IN — lowering the legs back to their position in Movement 1.
4. BREATHE OUT — finally lowering your legs back to the floor as in the starting position.
Repeat these sequence movements once again.

*Extension movements*
Don't forget to revert back to your normal breathing pattern.
1. Raise your feet until they are about twelve inches from the floor. Cross your right leg over your left, as far to the left as you can take it. Now uncross your legs.
2. Raise your legs into the air until they are perpendicular. Open the legs wide apart, then close them together again.
3. Lower your legs back to their position in Movement 1, but this time cross the left leg over the right, and take it as far to the right as you can. Then uncross your legs.
4. Lower both legs back to the floor, and into your starting position. Now relax completely.
Repeat the full Extension Movements once again.

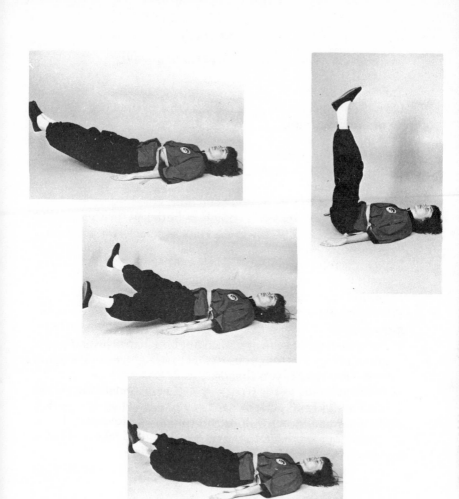
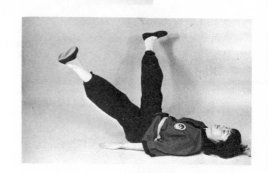

*Exercise 20    Willow Tree Stance (Liu Shu Shih)*

*Starting position*
Lie flat on the floor on your back, with legs stretched out and hands by your sides.

*Sequence movements*
1. BREATHE IN — raising both legs into the air, until they are perpendicular.
2. BREATHE OUT — as you bend both knees.
3. BREATHE IN — as you straighten both legs.
4. BREATHE OUT — lowering your legs back to the starting position.
Repeat the total sequence once again.

*Extension movements*
With normal breathing continuing throughout all the extension movements.
1. As Sequence Movement 1, then put both hands behind your knees, and pull hard as you attempt to straighten both of your legs. Then release your hands.
2. Put your hands on the front of your knees, and as you try to bend both knees, push as hard as you can with your hands.
3. Put your hands on the floor and straighten your legs.
4. Lower your legs back to the starting position.
Repeat all extensions once more.

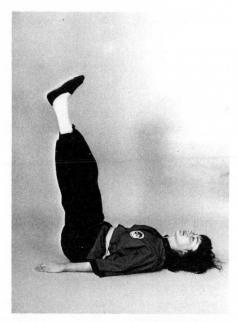

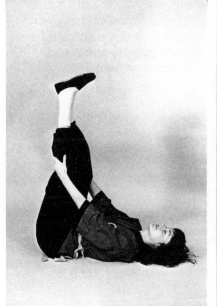

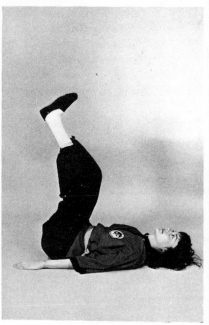

*Exercise 21    Willow Tree Stance (Liu Shu Shih)*

*Starting position*
As in Exercise 20.

*Sequence movements*
1. BREATHE IN — as you raise your body and legs perpen-dicularly into the air, putting your hands on your waist, so that your weight is supported on your hands and upper arms.
2. BREATHE OUT — and open the legs slightly, the left leg moving forward, the right leg moving backwards.
3. BREATHE IN — as you bring your legs together again.
4. BREATHE OUT — and open the legs slightly once more, but this time move the right leg forward and the left leg backward.
5. BREATHE IN — as you bring both legs together again.
6. BREATHE OUT — lowering your body and legs back onto the floor, and placing your arms by your sides.
Repeat this whole sequence once more.

*Extension movements*
Don't forget to keep your breathing as normal as you can.
1. As Sequence Movement 1.
2. As Sequence Movement 2, but this time try and open the legs as wide as possible, endeavouring to get both legs parallel to the floor with special attention to your right leg.
3. As Sequence Movement 3.
4. As Sequence Movement 4, with right leg forward and left leg back and opening the legs as wide as possible. Pay particular attention to the angle of the rear leg, getting it as low as you can.
5. As Sequence Movement 5.
6. As Sequence Movement 6.
Repeat all the Extension Movements again.

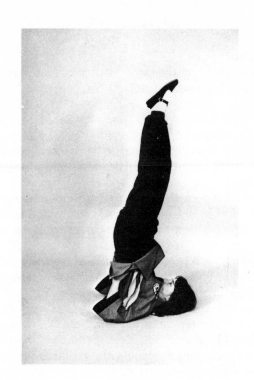

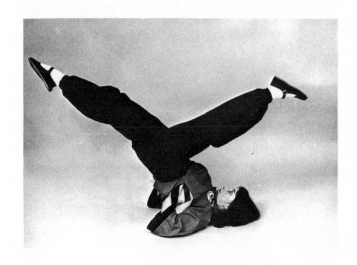

*Exercise 22    Cobra Stance (Yenching Shih)*

*Starting position*
Lie flat on your front on the floor, with your legs stretched out
behind you, and with your arms bent and held close by the sides
of the chest.

*Sequence movements*
1. BREATHE IN — as you point your toes directly to the rear,
   and at the same time lift your head so that your eyes look
   straight ahead.
2. BREATHE OUT — as you lower your head so that your chin
   rests on the floor, and let your body relax completely.
Repeat this sequence of movements two more times.

*Extension movements*
Once again, let us stress that during the Extension Movements
all breathing should be as normal as possible.
1. Point your toes directly to the rear, and raise your chest off
   the floor by straightening both arms; then slowly draw your
   head back as far as you can. Keep as much of your body as
   possible in continuous contact with the floor.
2. Lower your body and head back to the floor, and allow your
   arms to bend so that they return to their original starting
   position. Allow the body to relax completely.
Make a dual repetition of these Extension Movements.

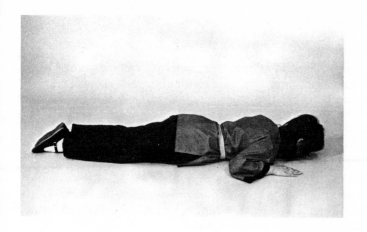

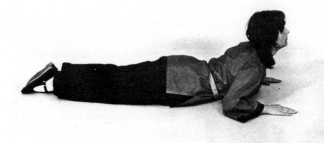

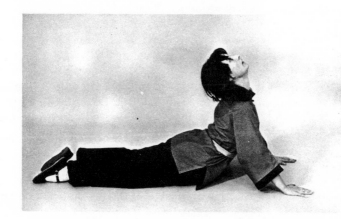

*Exercise 23    Fish Stance (Yu Shih)*

*Starting position*
Lie on your right side, fully stretched out, and bend your right
arm so as to support your head with your right hand. Left arm
laying on your left side.

*Sequence movements*
1. BREATHE IN — as you put your left hand on the floor in
   front of your chest.
2. BREATHE OUT — as you raise your left leg sideways into
   the air.
3. BREATHE IN — as you return the left leg to the starting
   position.
4. BREATHE OUT — as you roll over onto your back, then
   continue the roll so you finally go on to your left side, with
   full support for your head with your left hand, and your right
   arm laying on your right side.
5. BREATHE IN — whilst putting your right arm on the floor in
   front of your chest.
6. BREATHE OUT — as you raise your right leg sideways into
   the air.
7. BREATHE IN — on returning the right leg to the starting
   position.
8. BREATHE OUT — as you roll over completely back to your
   right side with your right arm supporting your head, and
   your left arm laying alongside your left hip and thighs.
Repeat this complete sequence of eight movements again.

*Extension movements*
Normal breathing during the extensions.
1. As Sequence Movement 1.
2. As Sequence Movement 2, but raise the left leg into the air as
   high as possible, and simultaneously raising your right hip
   and thigh off the floor by pushing strongly downward with
   right elbow, left hand, and the side of your right foot.
3. Return left leg and body to starting position.
4. As Sequence Movement 4.
5. As Sequence Movement 5.
6. As Sequence Movement 6, whilst you raise your right leg high

into the air, also lift your left hip and thigh off the floor, through the use of your left elbow, right hand, and the side of your left foot.

7. As Sequence Movement 7.
8. As Sequence Movement 8.

Go through all the Extension Movements once again.

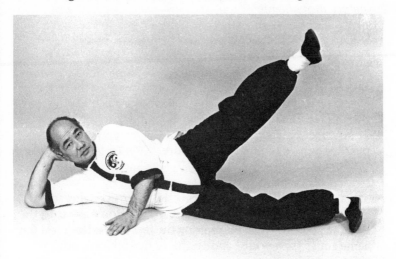

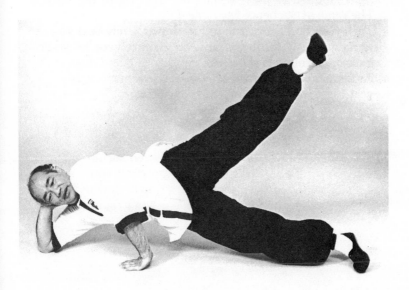

*Exercise 24    Eagle Stance (Tiao Shih)*

*Starting position*
Stand upright with both feet together, and your hands hanging
loosely by your sides.

*Sequence movements*
1. BREATHE IN — turning your body slowly to the right, and
   letting your arms swing with the turn of the body.
2. BREATHE OUT — as you turn your body back to the front,
   and allow your arms to return to your sides.
3. BREATHE IN — as this time you turn slowly to the left, and
   letting your arms swing with the turn of your body.
4. BREATHE OUT — turning your body back to the front with
   your arms returning to your sides.
Repeat the whole sequence once more.

*Extension movements*
As usual — normal breathing during the Extension Movements.
1. As Sequence Movement 1, but turn your body as far to the
   right as you can, without moving the feet on the floor. At the
   same time, turn your head to the right and look over your
   right shoulder.
2. The same as Sequence Movement 2.
3. Turn your body and arms as far round to the left as you can,
   simultaneously turning your head to the left so that you can
   look over your left shoulder.
4. As Sequence Movement 4.
Repeat these four Extension Movements again.

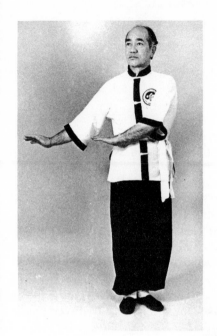

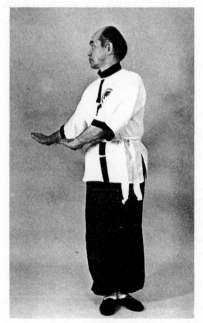

*Exercise 25    Eagle Stance (Tiao Shih)*

*Starting position*
As in Exercise 24.

*Sequence movements*
1. BREATHE IN — as you drop your head forward, so that you are looking down.
2. BREATHE OUT — whilst you roll your head 180 degrees to the right, and then back.
3. BREATHE IN — as you continue your head roll round to the left and back to the front, and you end up with your head looking down at your feet.
4. BREATHE OUT — as you straighten your head, so that you look directly ahead.
5. BREATHE IN — as you again drop your head forward, so that you look down.
6. BREATHE OUT — as you now roll your head round to the right, and then back, so that you have completed 180 degrees of the circle.
7. BREATHE IN — as you complete the circle with your head by allowing it to continue to the right and then to your front, so that you finish the circle looking down at your feet.
8. BREATHE OUT — as you raise your head to the starting position.
Repeat once more, circling the head to the right and then to the left.

*Extension movements*
Your normal breathing is required.
1. As Sequence Movement 1.
2. As Sequence Movement 2, but try and touch your right shoulder with your right cheek; then when going back try to put your head in between your shoulder blades.
3. As Sequence Movement 3, but endeavouring to touch your left shoulder with your left cheek, and when you get to the front, press your chin downward into your chest.
4. As Sequence Movement 4.
5. As Sequence Movement 5.
6. As Extension Movement 2, but in the reverse direction.

7. As Extension Movement 3, but continuing to the right.
8. As Sequence Movement 8.
Repeat all Extension Movements, but reverse the starting direction.

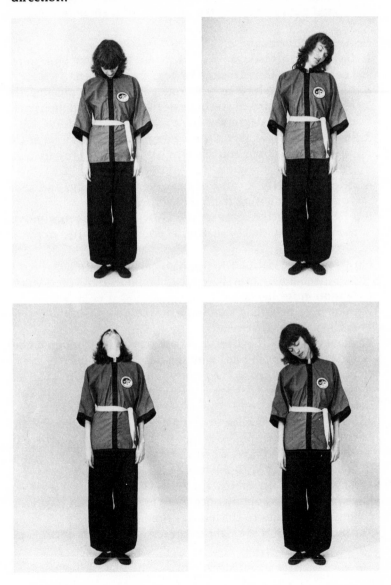

*Exercise 26    Bear Stance (Hsiung Shih)*

*Starting position*
Stand erect, looking directly ahead, with your hands by your sides, and your feet about the width of your shoulders apart.

*Sequence movements*
1. BREATHE IN — as you put your hands on your hips, keeping your thumbs close to your index fingers.
2. BREATHE OUT — as you roll your hips by pushing the abdomen forward, then continue to the right, and then back, completely 180 degrees of the circle.
3. BREATHE IN — as you now complete the full circle of the hips by rolling them round to the left, and finally round to the front again.
4. BREATHE OUT — as you straighten your body, and relax your arms by letting them return to your sides.
5-6-7-8. Exactly the same as the above four sequence movements, except that you rotate your hips in the opposite direction.
Now repeat the eight Sequence Movements once again.

*Extension movements*
Reminder — breathing should be normal.
1. As Sequence Movement 1.
2. As Sequence Movement 2, except that as the abdomen goes forward you push hard with the base of your palms; and as you roll your hips to the right you push hard with your left hand. As you move backwards then you pull hard with your fingers.
3. Still pulling hard with your fingers, you now continue the circling movement of your hips to the left, pushing hard with your right hand, and when getting back to the front again, once more push with the heel of the palms.
4. As Sequence Movement 4, and relax.
Repeat this circling action once more for 5-6-7-8, but start your rolling of your hips to the left this time.
Repeat the whole of the eight Extension Movements once again.

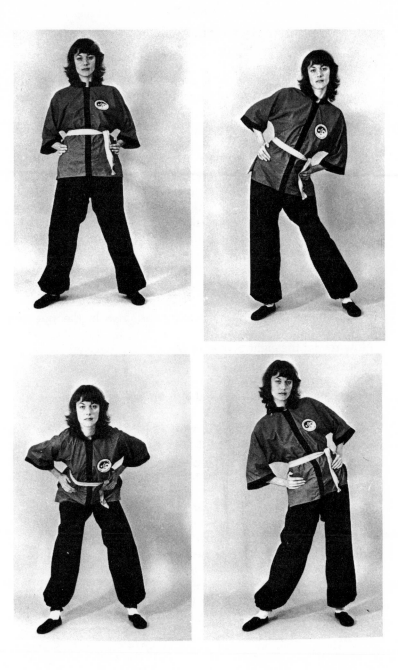

*Exercise 27    Bear Stance (Hsiung Shih)*

*Starting position*
As in Exercise 26.

*Sequence movements*
1. BREATHE IN — as you swing your arms backwards and then upwards so that your fingers point to the ceiling.
2. BREATHE OUT — as you now continue the swing on your arms forwards and downwards, trying to touch your toes. Keep both knees locked all the time. If you cannot touch your toes, then reach as far as you can, but do not bend the knees.
3. BREATHE IN — as you straighten your body, and your arms going back to your sides.
4. BREATHE OUT — as you relax within yourself.
Repeat the full sequence once more.

*Extension movements*
Because you are bending your body quite tightly you may find that retaining your normal breathing will be quite difficult — but try.
1. As Sequence Movement 1.
2. As Sequence Movement 2, but instead of touching your toes try to grip under your toes with your fingers. If you cannot do this to start with, then grip your leg or your ankle. Without bending the knees, step forward a little with your right foot, and follow this with your left foot.
3. Again without bending your knees, step back with your right foot, and then with your left foot. You should now be back in the starting position.
4. Release your grips, stand upright and allow your hands to go back to your sides, and relax.
Repeat the full Extension Movements, but changing "right" for "left" and *vice versa*.

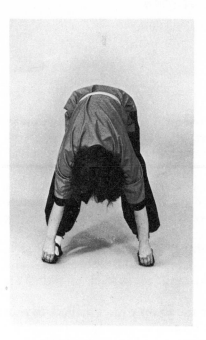

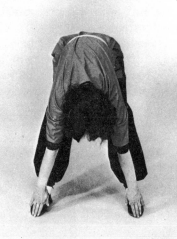

*Exercise 28    Leopard Stance (Pao Shih)*

*Starting position*
As in Exercise 26.

*Sequence movements*
1. BREATHE IN — raising your arms sideways until they are on
   a level with your shoulders, and at the same time bend your
   left knee, so that most of your body weight rests on your left
   leg.
2. BREATHE OUT — as you bend your body to the right, as
   you push your hips out to the left. Allow your left arm to
   swing over your head, while the right hand touches the
   outside of your right knee.
3. BREATHE IN — as you straighten your body and hips and
   bringing your weight evenly on both legs, and
   simultaneously letting your arms move back until they are
   level with the shoulders.
4. BREATHE OUT — whilst you lower your arms back to your
   sides.
5-6-7-8. Continue the above sequence but substitute "left" for
"right" and *vice versa.*
Now repeat the whole eight Sequence Movements once more.

*Extension movements*
Retain your normal breathing throughout the following
extensions.
1. As Sequence Movement 1.
2. As Sequence Movement 2, but as you bend sideways allow
   the fingers of your right hand to continue to slide down your
   right leg until the fingertips touch the floor or reach as low as
   you can get them.
3. As Sequence Movement 3.
4. As Sequence Movement 4.
5-6-7-8 is the continuation of these four extensions but now you
   change "left" to "right" and *vice versa.*
For the full benefit run through these eight extensions once
more.

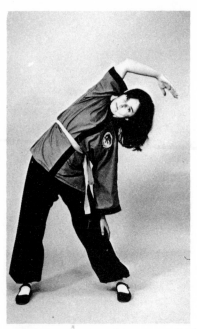

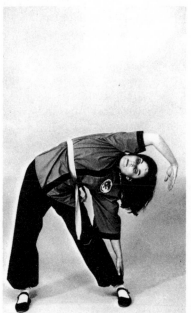

*Exercise 29     Leopard Stance (Pao Shih)*

*Starting position*
As in Exercise 26.

*Sequence movements*
1. BREATHE IN — as you raise your arms sideways until they are level with your shoulders, and at the same time bend your left knee and transfer most of your body weight on to your left leg.
2. BREATHE OUT — as you turn your head and look at your left hand.
3. BREATHE IN — as you turn your head back to the front.
4. BREATHE OUT — as you turn your head and look at your right hand.
5. BREATHE IN — as you turn your head back to the front.
6. BREATHE OUT — whilst you straighten your body, transfer your weight evenly on both legs, and lower both arms back to your sides.
Repeat the sequence, changing "left" to "right" and *vice versa*.

*Extension movements*
Breathing should be normal.
1. As Sequence Movement 1.
2. As Sequence Movement 2, but, after having turned your head to look at your hand, bend your head forward and try to look under your left armpit, and at the same time rotating your wrists so that your fingertips point down to the floor.
3. Lift your head so that it faces to the front again, and unwind your wrists so you are back into Movement 1.
4. The same as Sequence Movement 4, but once again, having turned your head to look to the right dip your head forward so that you can see under your right armpit, and simultaneously rotate your wrists again so that your fingers point downwards to the floor.
5. Unwind your wrists and lift your head so that it faces the front again.
6. As Sequence Movement 6.
Repeat once more but change "left" to "right" and *vice versa*.

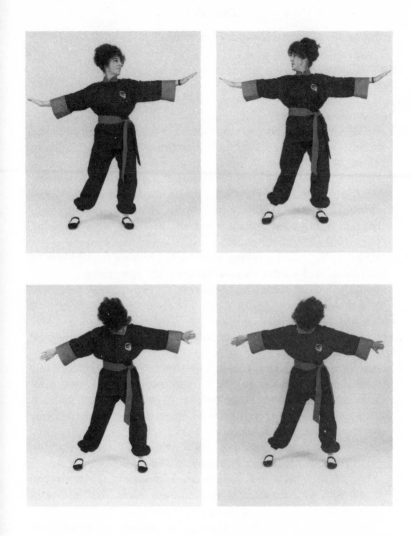

*Exercise 30    Leopard Stance (Pao Shih)*

*Starting position*
As in Exercise 26.

*Sequence movements*
1. BREATHE IN — as you step sideways with your left foot and bend your left knee, and let your arms swing to the right, to about waist height.
2. BREATHE OUT — bringing your left leg back to the starting position, and allow your arms to drop to your sides.
3. BREATHE IN — whilst you step sideways with your right foot, bending your right knee, and allow your arms to swing to the left, to waist height.
4. BREATHE OUT — taking your right leg back to the starting position, and letting your arms drop by your sides.
Repeat the full sequence once more.

*Extension movements*
Your normal breathing pattern should be maintained during the extensions.
1. As Sequence Movement 1, but the extra little bit on this exercise is that once having moved into position, you now also bend your right knee so that it touches the floor, but make sure that your right foot is kept in contact with the floor from heel to toe.
2. Straighten your right leg, then proceed to the starting position as in Sequence Movement 2.
3. This is the same as Extension Movement 1, with the exception, of course, that you change "right" to "left" and *vice versa*.
4. As Extension Movement 2, but change "left to "right" and *vice versa*.
Repeat these four Extension Movements once more.

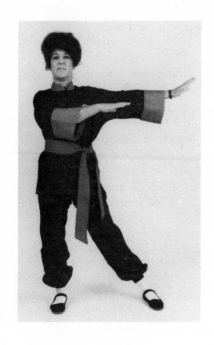

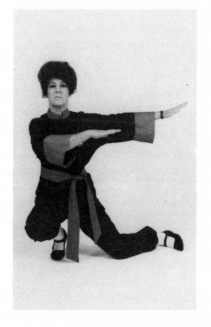

*Exercise 31    Riding Horse Stance (Ch'i Ma Shih)*

*Starting position*
Stand with feet together and arms hanging loosely by the thighs.

*Sequence movements*
1. BREATHE IN — as you step directly sideways with your left
   foot and bend your knees so that the thighs are almost parallel
   with the floor.
2. BREATHE OUT — raising your arms directly in front of your
   chest, until they are on a level with your shoulders.
3. BREATHE IN — lowering your arms to your sides, and
   straighten both legs.
4. BREATHE OUT — bringing your left foot back to the
   starting position.
5-8. Repeat the four Sequence Movements, but changing "left"
   to "right" and *vice versa*.
Now run through the whole eight Sequence Movements once
again.

*Extension movements*
Breathing should be normal during these extensions.
1. As Sequence Movement 1.
2. Don't stop your arms on a level with your shoulders, but
   allow the arms to continue upwards until your fingers point
   to the ceiling, and at the same time, bend your knees more
   deeply, by dropping your buttocks down to a position as
   close to the floor as you can.
3. As Sequence Movement 3.
4. As Sequence Movement 4.
5-8. Repeat the above Extension Movements once more but
   change "left" to "right" and *vice versa*.
Now repeat these eight Extension Movements once more.

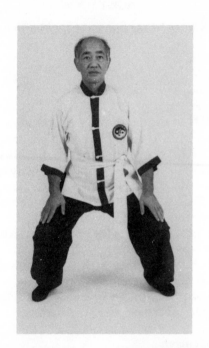

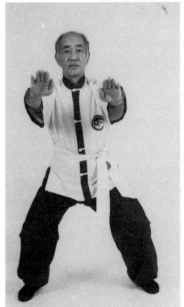

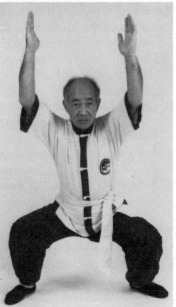

*Exercise 32    Riding Horse Stance (Ch'i Ma Shih)*

*Starting position*
As in Exercise 31.

*Sequence movements*
1. BREATHE IN — step sideways with your left foot and bend both knees.
2. BREATHE OUT — swing your arms directly backwards.
3. BREATHE IN — swing your arms directly forward until they are on a level with your shoulders.
4. BREATHE OUT — now bend forward so that your fingertips touch the ground in front of you.
5. BREATHE IN — straighten the body and also straighten both legs, and let your arms drop by your sides.
6. BREATHE OUT — bring your left foot back alongside your right foot, as in the starting position.
7-12. Now repeat the whole sequence once more, changing "left" to "right" and *vice versa*.

*Extension movements*
Breathing normal during these extensions.
1. As Sequence Movement 1.
2. Swing your arms directly backward and then slowly raise them behind your back as high as possible, and at the same time moving your head backwards so that you eventually look at the ceiling.
3. Now straighten the head, and at the same time let your arms swing directly forward until they are on a level with your shoulders.
4. Let your head droop forward as you deeply bend your body, simultaneously, let your arms swing on the insides of the legs, so that your hands curl round, and grip your ankles from the rear. Then pull your shoulders downwards as much as possible.
5. As Sequence Movement 5.
6. As Sequence Movement 6.
7-12. Repeat the above extensions, but change "left" to "right" and *vice versa*.

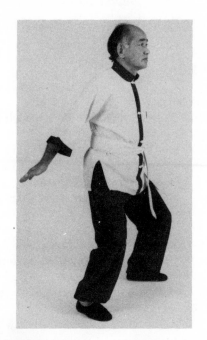

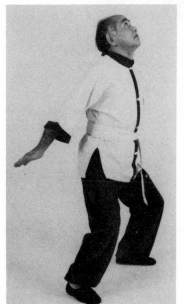

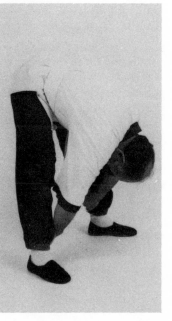

*Exercise 33   Leg Triangle Stance (T'ui Sanchiao Shih)*

*Starting position*
As in Exercise 31.

*Sequence movements*
1. BREATHE IN — step directly to the left with your left foot, and keep both legs straight.
2. BREATHE OUT — bend forward and touch the toes of your left foot with the fingertips of both hands.
3. BREATHE IN — keeping the fingertips of your left hand touching the toes of your left foot, move your right hand to the right so that the fingertips touch the toes of your right foot.
4. BREATHE OUT — keeping the fingertips of your right hand touching the toes of your right foot, swing your left arm over to the right so that the fingertips of your left hand are also touching the toes of your right foot.
5. BREATHE IN — relax and stand erect.
6. BREATHE OUT — bring your left foot back to the starting position.
7-12. Repeat the above sequence, but change "left" to "right" and *vice versa*.

*Extension movements*
Keep breathing normally during the extensions.
These are the same as the Sequence Movements, except that instead of touching your toes with your fingertips you place the palms of your hands on the floor just in front of your toes, keeping your knees locked and your legs straight.

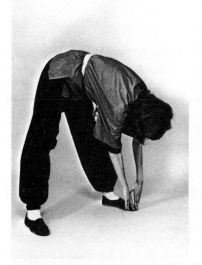
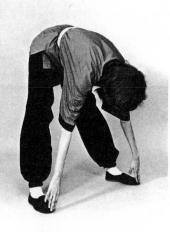
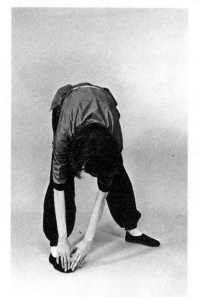
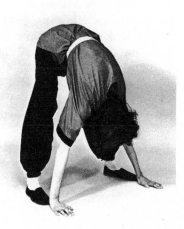

*Exercise 34    Leg Triangle Stance (T'ui Sanchiao Shih)*

*Starting position*
As in Exercise 31.

*Sequence movements*
1. BREATHE IN — step directly to the left with your left foot,
   and at the same time raise your arms sideways until they are
   level with your shoulders.
2. BREATHE OUT — bend downwards and outwards to your
   right, placing the fingers of your left hand on the floor beyond
   the toes of your right foot. Keep your legs straight, and the
   right arm moves naturally with the turn of the shoulders.
3. BREATHE IN — straighten the body, keeping your arms
   level with your shoulders.
4. BREATHE OUT — as you lower your arms back to your
   sides, and more your left foot back to the starting position.
5-8. Execute the above sequence again, but substitute "left" for
   "right" and *vice versa*.
Repeat the complete set of eight Sequence Movements once
more.

*Extension movements*
Normal breathing pattern during the extensions.
1. As Sequence Movement 1.
2. As Sequence Movement 2, but also turn your head so that
   you look up at the fingers of your right hand.
3. As Sequence Movement 3.
4. As Sequence Movement 4.
5-8. Execute the above extension again, but change "left" to
   "right" and *vice versa*.
Now repeat once more the complete extensions from 1 to 8.

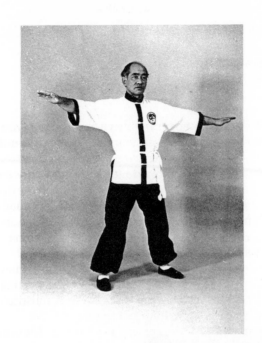

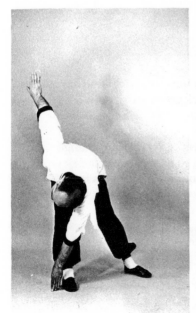

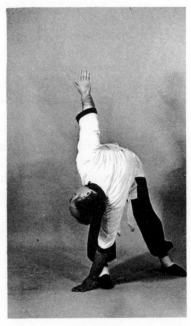

*Exercise 35    Dragon Stance (Lung Shih)*

*Starting position*
As in Exercise 31.

*Sequence movements*
1. BREATHE IN — step forward a pace and a half with your left foot, putting most of your weight onto it and bending your left knee. At the same time, swing your arms directly forward and upward until they are on a level with your shoulders. The back leg should be straight.
2. BREATHE OUT — whilst transferring your body weight onto your right leg, bending your right knee, and straightening your left leg. At the same time swing both arms downward and then backward until your hands are to the rear of your body, and bend your body forward.
3. BREATHE IN — as you straighten your body and allow your arms to drop down by your sides.
4. BREATHE OUT — withdrawing your left foot back to the starting position.
5-8. Repeat the sequence changing "left" to "right" and *vice versa*.
Now repeat the whole eight Sequence Movements once more.

*Extension movements*
Breathing normal, during the extension movements.
1. As Sequence Movement 1, but move your arms over the top of your head, leaning back as far as possible. Keeping your weight on the front leg.
2. As Sequence Movement 2, bending your body as far forward as you can and at the same time move your head downward towards your front knee. The arms, continue their swing, in an upward and forward direction as far as possible.
3. As Sequence Movement 3.
4. As Sequence Movement 4.
5-8. Execute the extensions once again but reverse the stance.
Now repeat all the Extension Movements once more.

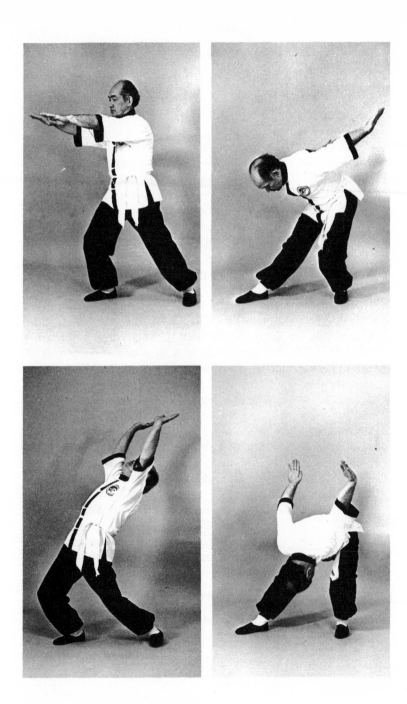

*Exercise 36    Crossed-Leg Stance (Ch'iao Cho T'ui Shih)*

*Starting position*
As in Exercise 31.

*Sequence movements*
1. BREATHE IN — cross your right leg in front of your left leg, with the toes of your right foot just touching the floor.
2. BREATHE OUT — bring your right leg back to the starting position.
3. BREATHE IN — cross your left leg in front of your right leg, with the toes of your left foot just touching the floor.
4. BREATHE OUT — bring your left leg back to the starting position.
5-8. Repeat the above four Sequence Movements.

*Extension movements*
Retain your normal breathing during the following extensions.
1. Carry out Sequence Movement 1, then raise your arms sideways until they are on a level with your shoulders and lift your chest as high as possible. At the same time lower your right heel to the floor, so that the back of your right knee presses firmly against the front of your left knee.
2. Return your right leg and your arms back to the starting position.
3. As Extension Movement 1, but change "right" to "left" and *vice versa*.
4. Return to the starting position.

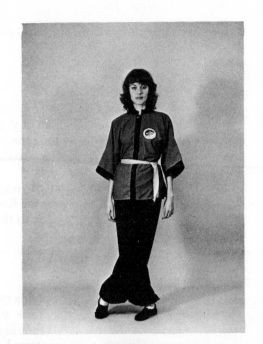

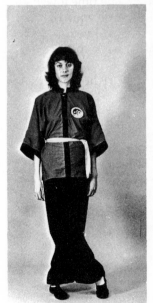

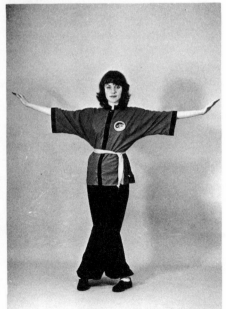

*Exercise 37    Crossed-Leg Stance (Ch'iao Cho T'ui Shih)*

*Starting position*
As in Exercise 31.

*Sequence movements*
1. BREATHE IN — cross your right leg in front of your left leg,
   with the toes of your right foot just touching the floor. At the
   same time raise your arms sideways until they are on a level
   with your shoulders.
2. BREATHE OUT — as you slowly return to the starting
   position.
3. BREATHE IN — cross your left leg in front of your right leg,
   with the toes of the left foot just touching the floor. At the
   same time raise your arms sideways until they are both on a
   level with your shoulders.
4. BREATHE OUT — uncross your legs, and lower your arms
   and return to the starting position.
5-8. Repeat these four Sequence Movements.

*Extension movements*
Maintain your normal breathing.
1. As Sequence Movement 1.
2. Rest your body weight on the toes of your right foot, and turn
   your left foot onto its side. Move your body weight back on
   to your left leg and turn your right foot on to its side on the
   floor.
3. Return to the starting position.
4. As Sequence Movement 3.
5. As Extension Movement 2, but change "right" for "left" and
   *vice versa*.
6. Resume the starting position.
7-12. Duplicate the above Extension Movements once more.

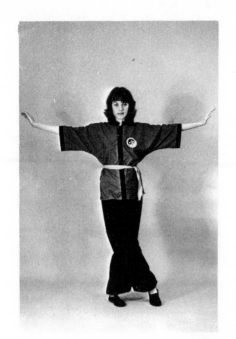

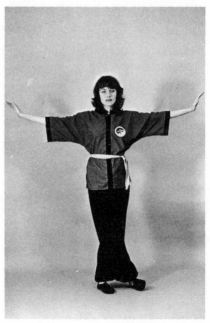

*Exercise 38   Scissor Stance (Chien Tao Shih)*

*Starting position*
As in Exercise 31.

*Sequence movements*
1. BREATHE IN — rest your weight on your left leg, and move
   your right foot behind and beyond your left foot. At the same
   time raise both arms sideways until they are on a level with
   your shoulders. Bend your knees so that your right knee
   touches the middle of your left calf.
2. BREATHE OUT — as you slowly straighten both legs and
   resume the starting position.
3. BREATHE IN — as you execute Movement 1, but change
   "left" to "right" and *vice versa*.
4. BREATHE OUT — whilst you straighten your legs and
   resume the starting position.
5-8. Repeat the above sequences once more.

*Extension movements*
Remember to maintain your normal breathing for the
extensions.
The Extension Movements for this exercise are the same as the
sequence, except that you bend the knee of the rear leg till it
touches the heel of the front foot.

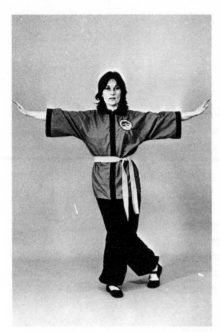

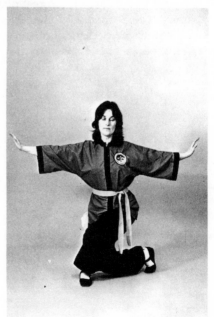

*Exercise 39    Monkey Stance (Hou Shih)*

*Starting position*
As in Exercise 31.

*Sequence movements*
1. BREATHE IN — step back one pace with your left foot, placing most of your body weight on your left leg, and bending your left knee.
2. BREATHE OUT — let your arms swing forward and upward until they are on a level with your shoulders.
3. BREATHE IN — transfer your weight onto your right leg, and lift your right heel off the floor, so that the toes are taking the weight. Simultaneously let your arms swing back.
4. BREATHE OUT — step forward with your left foot and resume the starting position.
5-8.  Repeat the sequence, but change "left" to "right" and *vice versa*.

*Extension movements*
Let your breathing remain completely normal.
Same as the Sequence Movements, but the extension is created by the simple expedient of pushing down hard on the foot that is taking the weight of the body.

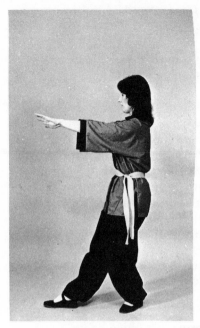

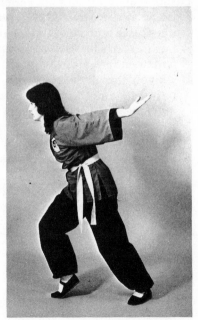

*Exercise 40    Chicken Stance (Hsiao Chi Shih)*

*Starting position*
Stand erect with your hands by your thighs and your feet a little wider than the width of your shoulders apart.

*Sequence movements*
1. BREATHE IN — turning the whole of your body to the left, pivoting on the ball of each foot. Keeping your body erect, bend your right knee until it is about an inch from the floor.
2. BREATHE OUT — straighten your legs and turn back so that you face the front once more.
3. BREATHE IN — turning the whole of your body to the right, pivoting on the ball of each foot. Keeping your body erect, bend your left knee until it is about an inch from the floor.
4. BREATHE OUT — straighten your legs and turn back so that you face the front once more.
5-8. Repeat these Sequence Movements once more.

*Extension movements*
Ensure that you retain your normal breathing habits.
1. As Sequence Movement 1, but after having bent your right knee place both hands on top of your left thigh, and lean your head back as far as possible, and at the same time push your abdomen forward.
2. As you straighten your legs, push strongly downwards on both legs, and this will help you to raise yourself. Then turn and face the front, as in your starting position.
3. As Sequence Movement 3, but after having bent your left knee place both hands on top of your right thigh, and lean your head back as far as possible, and push your abdomen forward.
4. Straighten your legs, pushing yourself up with both hands, and then turn and face the front, as in the starting position.

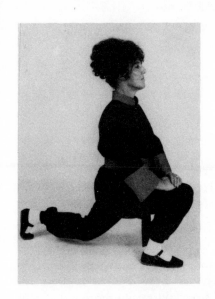

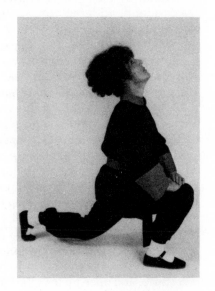

## Chapter 9

# Meditation

Although many people have gone to great lengths in an effort to learn how to meditate, and yet have been disappointed, meditation is easy provided that you go into it for the right reasons, and, with the help of a good master or teacher, look into it thoroughly, so that you learn the basics of what is involved, become clear about your own objectives, and then set out under guidance in an effort to achieve them. A good teacher will make sure that you take each step properly, at the right speed for you, and that you develop a proper understanding.

First of all, to get to the spirit you must go through the mind, and to get to the mind you must go along the channels of your earthly body. You must be prepared for a long journey of the spirit, and have ample supplies of the energies required — just as a car or an aeroplane needs fuel. Remember that in meditating you are going to use up an enormous amount of physical, mental and spiritual energy, even though your journey may last only a few minutes as measured by the hands of a clock. For this reason, one of your prime tasks is to build up your energies, helping along the process by eating the Ch'ang Ming way (see Chapter 4) so as to reduce the excess of Yin that other types of diet cause, and open up the internal channels of the body so that your internal energy can flow properly. K'ai Men and the various deep-breathing exercises recommended in Chapter 5 (especially the Yang exercises) help to build up this energy in the Tan T'ien or lower abdomen. As you progress you will be able to utilize this energy and control it at various levels in your body, so developing heightened mental control as well. This leads on to spiritual growth.

After adopting a Ch'ang Ming diet and learning how to cultivate your internal energy, the next step is to learn how to harness and control your macro-cosmic, or external, energy. When your internal and external energy can be harmonized at a point behind your eyes, then you will find consciousness an easy stepping-stone to awareness, and enlightenment will be just round the corner.

There are over twenty forms of Taoist meditation (Mo Hsiang), but to practise them you must be able to direct and control your internal and external energies, which will give you the dynamic power that you need if you want to traverse the universe. This force also has enormous healing powers.

One of the easiest ways of starting to meditate is to sit quietly down — if possible, at the same time each day — in a room where you can expect no disturbance. Have a window slightly open so that fresh air can enter the room, but try to ensure that there are no draughts. You can sit on a chair or cross your legs on the floor, or you can sit in the lotus position, which is the ideal way to meditate as it ensures perfect balance. In what follows it is assumed that you decide to sit cross-legged on the floor.

Loosen your clothes, especially any belts, and then relax your whole body and mind. Sit with your left leg crossed outside, but close to, your right leg — signifying that the Yin is surrounding the Yang. Your left hand should be placed in the palm of your right hand, with the left thumb touching the middle finger of the left hand, and the right thumb laid flat in the centre of the left palm. The palms of both hands should face upward. This ensures that the Yang surrounds the Yin in the upper circle of the body. By sitting this way, you are embracing the eight psychic channels and centres of the body, four in the lower half and four in the upper half of your anatomy. These circles or circuits create a harmony, and a constant flow of energy within their own individual orbits.

Before commencing to meditate make absolutely certain that you have no emotional stress whatsoever, and that you feel completely calm and composed within yourself. Also be certain that you have no aches or pains, as these can upset your concentration. It is not a good thing to set a goal or target for yourself, as this encourages you to try too hard. Try not to be too specific in your reasons for meditating, since this tends to create emotion and upset the nervous system. Many people try to meditate to obtain peace and tranquillity, while others wish to meditate just to escape from this world and the realities of their own lives — forgetting, of course, that on awakening they will be back in the same situations as they had tried to forget or leave behind. Meditation should not be an excuse, but should be a serious endeavour to attain harmony with your own spirit and, through it, with the spiritual world that lies beyond.

There are many ways of meditating with the eyes closed, but you can also meditate with your eyes open. Further, you can meditate not only through the mind but also through the spirit. One form of meditation, visual transportation, enables people to meditate through their eyes, mind and spirit, while they go about their daily work.

A golden rule for beginners to remember is that one should not stare at objects for long periods ("meditation by focusing"). It is much better to concentrate the mind, with the eyes closed, than to stare at a lighted candle, because the latter can not only weaken the eyes and waste energy, which in the preparatory stages you should be trying to conserve, but also mislead the senses into a false sense of achievement.

To begin with, then, sit quietly in the cross-legged position described above, with your tongue against the roof of your mouth and your eyes fractionally open (sufficient to admit a thin film of light) and looking down the bridge of your nose. Next concentrate your mind on whatever object you wish, and, when you have it in focus, keep it in your mind's eye for as long as you can.

Let us suppose that you fix your mind on an old-fashioned sailing ship. Once you have formed the picture, begin examining it in detail. How many masts are there? Is there a figurehead at the prow, and, if so, what is its form? Where is the anchor? Are the hatches battened down?

While you are still at the elementary stage, never meditate for more than five minutes at a time. This is because deep concentration uses up energy, and it is unwise to burn up a lot of "fuel" while you are still trying to activate and cultivate the energies within you. Once you have managed to focus your mind on one object for five minutes, the next step is to explore other forms of mind control and concentration.

Focusing on sound is difficult, but will give you a very strong mind control. If you are sitting quietly you will hear noises and sounds going on around you all the time, and if you concentrate enough you will be able to pick out one of those sounds (the most prominent, say) and hold it in your mind, making all other sounds disappear. Once you have learned to eradicate all other noises, and hold just one in your mind constantly, you will know that your mind is becoming very strong indeed.

Another, and even more difficult, way to meditate is to focus on smell. Bring in a pot of flowers and place them directly in front of you, and then sit quietly in front of them, breathing deeply. Learn to focus on the smell of one particular type of flower, so that other perfumes and smells fade away before it. In this way your concentration will gain enormous strength, and your mind will become extremely tenacious.

Remember that the journey for which you are preparing is a very long one, so it is essential that you prepare properly. Don't forget that correct breathing is essential to your meditation, so learn to breathe through the lower abdomen, as described in Chapter 5. This will help you build up your energies and gain tranquillity.

Everything in nature consists of energy, which in turn creates various wavelengths and vibrations; so to lack energy is in the long run fatal. Lack of energy creates fatigue, which is the basis of all illnesses and sicknesses. Revitalize the organ or section of the body that is fatigued and you eradicate the symptom, allowing the body to cure itself. In meditation, then, you must have the whole body active and full of energy, and all the channels open, so that the energy flow is unrestricted. Then you can really start to meditate seriously, for then the energy power is there to help the mind take full control and prepare for take-off. So get your priorities right and you will find that meditation is within your grasp.

If you happen to be a nervous person or a persistent worrier, then to begin with you should not try to meditate at all. Instead, concentrate on building up your vitality by eating the Ch'ang Ming way and practising deep-breathing exercises, and sit quietly for a few minutes daily, thinking, with your eyes open, of some material object — a door handle, a vase, a chair, or whatever — imagining its shape and contours, its colour, and even how it is made. After only a few weeks you will find that you have made great progress and are ready to focus your mind as suggested earlier.

Everyone who practises properly, should, after a few months, be able to journey into the astral plane, but travelling to the celestial and spiritual levels takes rather longer. Even so, with a good teacher, patience and personal dedication this can be accomplished by all.

Finally, take no notice of people who brag about their own feats of meditation. There is no place in the spiritual world for egoists, and whatever they experienced is unlikely to have been of much consequence.

Good travelling, and perhaps we may meet along the way.

## Chapter 10

# Healing

The Tao is the order and the way of everything in the universe, from the tiniest particle of dust to vast galaxies, and within the Tao is the balance and harmony of Yin and Yang, the Dual Monism of all things. You are part of this order, and any illness that you may suffer is brought on by internal imbalance and can be cured. Learn to harmonize with the rest of the universe, physically, mentally and spiritually, and do your utmost to help others.

Prevention is better than cure, and eating the Ch'ang Ming way (see Chapter 4) will keep sickness away from you. If, however, you are already suffering from something, then a Ch'ang Ming diet will help to eradicate that weakness, as the following testimonies by previous sufferers make clear (quotes from the Luton *Evening Post* of 1971):

*Mrs H. Ruff (Luton)*. "I had suffered from migraine for 19 years. They were always bad attacks with vomiting and stomach upsets. I used to spend two days in bed sometimes. The doctor would give me injections to put me out, there was nothing else he could do. I was finally having attacks every nine or ten days. Now I feel like I did in my teens. It's marvellous."

*Mrs J. Slow (Northampton)*. "I had multiple sclerosis for 23 years. Four years ago I was so bad I could hardly put one leg in front of the other, and after the last attack my hands were severely afflicted. I am now a ward orderly in a hospital, and enjoy it, and I have so much energy, and can run upstairs. The multiple sclerosis association in Northampton considers me the wonder girl."

*Mrs M. Chance (Limbury).* "I had arthritis for three years, and the doctors said there was nothing they could do, except give me tablets to kill the pain. Now I am much better and there is only the top joint to go. I know it takes time to cure, but I am better already."

*Mrs J. Peddar (Dunstable).* "I suffered from muscular rheumatism. This year was the first summer holiday in three years that I haven't suffered while I've been away."

*Mrs B. McIntyre (Luton).* "When I came first I just couldn't see straight. I'd had migraine attacks for four years. It was getting the family down. I've got three children aged six, four and two. I used to push them in a room and shut the door on them to try and get peace and quiet. Since I came here, I have not had an attack since. Now I can go out with the children."

These are just a few of thousands who have benefited from balancing the Yin and Yang within their bodies by Ch'ang Ming and by carrying out Taoist breathing exercises.

Practising K'ai Men is of enormous benefit to the health and also makes available to the practitioner the many potent Taoist methods of healing. The following are brief descriptions of some of them.

## Ch'i Healing

This is healing by use of the breath, which activates the internal energy and causes vibrations along the lines of meridian. Depending on the type of illness suffered, the breath can be altered so as to help correct the inbalance at the root of the trouble.

When you have acquired a deep understanding of the Yin and Yang methods of Taoist breathing, and have learnt how to control and pass on your internal energy, you will be able to channel some of this energy to anyone who needs it. You need not worry that you will thereby be depriving yourself, for by practising K'ai Men and eating the Ch'ang Ming way you will have energy to spare.

## Chentung Healing

This too is a form of vibration healing and utilizes the lines of meridian. The vibration is caused through sound waves, which can be adjusted so that they are able to modify the Yin and Yang. By making contact between two points along the lines of meridian, all the major organs can be activated.

## Li Healing

This makes use of macro-cosmic energy, which our bodies do not have to generate, since it is constantly passing through us. What we have to do is to learn how to harness, store and control it. The potential of macro-cosmic energy is astounding (see Chapter 2), and if you can harmonize it with your internal energy then your spiritual strength will be enormous and you will have the seeds of spiritual immortality within yourself.

Macro-cosmic energy, when used for healing purposes, can stop symptoms almost immediately. So learn to develop this energy to the full through practising K'ai Men, and you will be able to help and serve many people who are desperately in need of assistance.

## Ts'ao Pen Chih Wu Healing

This is basically herbal therapy. As has been outlined earlier, the ancient Chinese explored this field in very great depth, acquainting themselves with the properties of over 30,000 herbs, many of which are still widely used. In the sixteenth century a Chinese scientist, Lee Shi Tzen, wrote fifty-two books on the subject, after spending nearly thirty years studying it.

What is not widely realized is that the ancient Chinese also made a close study of the nutritional value of birds, animals, and fish and other seafood. Seahorses had an excellent reputation as a pick-me-up; lizards were often used in treatment for asthma and to help wounds heal more quickly; cuttlefish bones were used as an antacid, as they contain quite a powerful astringent; certain types of crab were used as antidotes to poison; and dried silkworms were used in treating epilepsy and angina. Today, however, these remedies are largely discontinued, as everything needed for helping the sick and suffering can be obtained from the plant world.

**Jeh Healing**
This is a form of heat treatment, making extensive use of compresses and helping to generate energy along the lines of meridian. Garlic, rice, mustard, ginger and moxa, as well as water, are among the substances used.

Both this and the other methods of healing outlined in this chapter will be learnt by anyone who makes sufficient progress in K'ai Men.

---

# The Chinese Cultural Arts Association

All the Taoist arts, such as Taoism, Taoist Yoga (K'ai Men), Taoist Philosophy, Taoist Healing, Taoist Meditation, and T'ai Chi Ch'uan and other accompanying arts were first introduced into England by a Chinese businessman, Professor Chan Lee, who in 1930 started the first club in London for those who wished to learn about these arts. Because of the war the club had to close in 1939, but it re-opened again in 1950 and shortly afterwards a second club was started in East London.

Stringent grading rules were laid down in 1951, and the Chinese Cultural Arts Association was formed so that all clubs and practitioners would be together under one banner. This has proved very successful, and many associated clubs have been formed, both in Britain and overseas.

Professor Chan Lee died in the winter of 1953-4, and it was natural that his nephew, Chee Soo, who had trained with him from the age of fourteen, should take over the leadership of the organization.

In 1958 Chee Soo set up the central coaching school, and laid down the rules and examinations for all coaches, from instructors to national coaches. These rules and examinations are still in force today, so standards are kept to a very high level. Anyone may apply to join local Teacher's training classes, which are held, generally for one day every two months, under the personal instruction of Chee Soo. Day courses can also be arranged with any class, club or groups of clubs.

Information on any subject concerning the Chinese Arts may be acquired from:

> The Chinese Cultural Arts Association,
> 426 Charter Avenue,
> Canley,
> Coventry CV4 8BD
> England.

# Index

Acceptance, 13, 25
Acupuncture, 10, 34
Alchemy
  physical, 11
  spiritual, 9
  Taoist, 23, 24, 46
Asthma, 43, 157

Bear stance (Hsiung
  Shih), 64, 120-3
Bodhidharma, 11, 12,
  60
Body, 30
Breathing, 14, 15, 16,
  31, 42-9, 57, 150,
  156
  yang, 46
  yin, 44
  yin/yang, 46-7
Bronchitis, 43

Ch'ang Ming diet, 14,
  24, 30, 33, 36-41,
  43, 54, 56-7, 59, 150,
  151, 153, 155, 156
Chan Lee, 33
Chentung healing, 157
Ch'i healing, 10, 34,
  49, 156
Chicken stance (Hsiao
  Chi Shih), 67, 148-9
Chinese Cultural Arts
  Association, 158

Chinese massage, 10
Christ, 11, 12, 24
Chuang Tzu, 11, 23
Cobra stance
  (Yenching Shih),
  63, 112-3
Concentration, 26-7
Confucius, 11
Cross-leg stance (Ch'iao
  Cho T'ui Shih), 68,
  140-3

Diet, see Ch'ang Ming
Double plough stance
  (Shuang Chang Li
  Shih), 61, 78-87
Dragon stance (Lung
  Shih), 65, 138-9
Drunkard stance (Tsui
  Han Shih), 62,
  100-107
Dual Monism, 10, 11,
  13, 17, 31, 33, 155

Eagle stance (Tiao
  Shih), 64, 116-9
Egoism, 25-6
Eight Strands of the
  Brocade, 56
Emphysema, 42-3
Energies, 9, 10, 15, 18,
  27, 28, 31, 34, 43,
  52, 150, 153

Exterior/external arts,
  12

Fish stance (Yu Shih),
  63, 114-5
Five elements (Wu
  Hsing), 31-2

Golden Stove (Chin
  Lu), see Lower stove

Healing, 31-4, 155-8;
  see also individual
  healing methods
Herbal therapy, 10, 33,
  34, 37, 157
Ho Hsien ('harmony'),
  see K'ai Men
Ho Ping ('unity'), see
  K'ai Men
Hypnotism, 16

Internal massage, see
  'Movement with
  stillness'
Inner Ch'i circling, 44
Internal arts, 12
Internal energy
  (Neichung Ch'i), 12,
  15-17, 34, 43, 44
Intrinsic energy (T'ien
  Jan Neng Li), see
  Internal energy

Jeh healing, 158

K'ai Men, 12, 13, 14,
    18, 20, 21, 27, 29,
    31, 34, 35, 37, 43,
    44, 47, 49, 56, 57,
    58, 59, 61, 150, 156,
    157, 158
    five doorways of,
    21
    postures and
    exercises, 20, 31,
    49, 60-7, 69-149;
    see also individual
    stances

Lao Tzu, 11, 18, 23
Law of Repercussion
    (Yin K'uo), 19
Lee Shi Tzen, 157
Leg triangle stance
    (T'ui Sanchiao
    Shih), 65, 134-7
Leopard stance (Pao
    Shih), 66, 124-9
Li healing, 10, 34, 157
Lines of meridian, 10,
    32, 34, 55
Lotus leaf stance (Ho
    Hua Yeh Shih), 62,
    88-91
Lower stove/cauldron
    (Hsia Lu), 16, 44,
    50

Macro-cosmic energy
    (Ching Sheng Li),
    10, 17-18, 24, 34,
    43, 157
Martial arts, 11-12
Meditation, 9, 10, 15,
    16, 17, 27-9, 150-4
    healing by, 32, 49
Mental energy, 15
Meridian healing, 10,
    49
Micro-cosmic energy,
    10

Mind, 24-9, 57-8
Monkey stance (Hou
    Shih), 66, 146-7
'Movement with
    stillness' (Yun Tung
    Pu Yun Tung), 60,
    69-149
Muscle changes, 14

Nei Ching, 34, 37

Outer Ch'i circle, 44

Physical energy, 14-15
Praying Mantis stance
    (Tao Lang Shih),
    63, 96-9
Psychic centres, 28, 43,
    52
Purification, 14, 15,
    24, 25, 30-1

Relaxation, 56
Revitalization, 14, 153
Riding Horse stance
    (Ch'i Ma Shih), 67,
    130-3

Scissor stance (Chien
    Tao Shih), 68, 144-5
Shaolin Temple, 11,
    12, 60
Single plough stance
    (Tan Chang Li
    Shih), 61, 70-7
Sleep, 53-4
Spirit, 22-4
Spiritual control, 18-20
Spiritual
    transportation
    (Ching Shen Yun
    Shu), 29
Stress, 26
Supreme Spirit, 11, 21,
    22, 23, 25, 26, 27,
    35, 59

T'ai Chi Ch'uan, 12,
    158
Talismans, 32
Tao, see Taoism
Taoism, 11, 12, 13, 16,
    19, 21, 22, 23, 24,
    25, 26, 29, 30, 32,
    33, 35, 59, 155
Taoist meditation (Mo
    Hsiang), see
    Meditation
Taoist yoga, see K'ai
    Men
Time, 18
Ts'ao Pen Chih Wu
    healing, see
    Herbal therapy
Turtle stance (Pie
    Shih), 64, 92-5

Visual transportation
    (Shih Li Yun Shu),
    29
Vitalities, see Energies
Vitality, 54-5
Vitality power (Sheng
    Ch'i), see
    Internal energy

Willow tree stance (Liu
    Shu Shih), 62,
    108-11

Yang breath, 50-1
Yang macro-cosmic
    circle, 44, 46
Yin and yang, 10, 11,
    13, 16, 17, 20, 22,
    29, 31, 32, 33, 34,
    35, 36, 37, 39, 43,
    44, 45, 46, 48-52
    passim, 54, 69,
    150, 151, 155, 157
Yin breath, 51-2, 56
Yin micro-cosmic
    orbit, 44, 46
Yin/yang breath, 52